Prentice-Hall Foundations of Speech Pathology Series

PRENTICE-HALL INTERNATIONAL, INC., *London*
PRENTICE-HALL OF AUSTRALIA, PTY., LTD., *Sydney*
PRENTICE-HALL OF CANADA, LTD., *Toronto*
PRENTICE-HALL OF INDIA (PRIVATE) LTD., *New Delhi*
PRENTICE-HALL OF JAPAN, INC., *Tokyo*
PRENTICE-HALL DE MEXICO, S.A., *Mexico City*

Cerebral Palsy

EUGENE T. MCDONALD

Research Professor
The Pennsylvania State University

BURTON CHANCE, JR.

Associate Surgeon
Orthopedic Department
The Children's Hospital of Philadelphia

ᘔᘔᘔ

Prentice-Hall, Inc., *Englewood Cliffs, N. J.*

editor's note

THE SET OF VOLUMES WHICH CONSTITUTES THE *Foundations of Speech Pathology* is designed to serve as the nucleus of a professional library, both for students of speech pathology and audiology and for the practicing clinician. Each individual text in the series is written by an author whose authority has long been recognized in his field. Each author has done his utmost to provide the basic information concerning the speech or hearing disorders covered in his book. Our new profession needs new tools, good ones, to be used not once but many times. The flood of new information already upon us requires organization if it is to help us solve the many different professional problems which beset us. This series provides that essential organization.

One of the unifying and outstanding features of all the volumes in this series is the use of search items. In addition to providing the core of information concerning his subject, each author has indicated clearly other sources having significance for the topic being discussed. The reader is urged to explore, to search, and to discover—and the trails are charted. In so rapidly changing a profession as ours, we cannot afford to remain content with what we have been taught. We must learn to continue learning.

Although each individual volume in this series is complete unto itself, the instructor should welcome the opportunity presented by the *Foundations of Speech Pathology* to combine several volumes to form the basic structure of the course he teaches. They may also be used as collateral readings. These short but comprehensive books give the instructor a thoroughly flexible teaching tool. But the primary aim of the authors of these texts has been the creation of a basic library for all of our students and professional workers. In this series we have sought to provide a common fund of knowledge to help unify and serve our new profession.

preface

A LARGE PROPORTION OF THE CEREBRAL PALSIED CHILDREN IN THE
United States receive their evaluations and treatments at the hands of
amateurs. The reader may object to this statement, pointing out that the
professional workers who see the children possess various degrees and
certificates. This is true, but only a few professional workers see enough
cerebral palsied patients and get enough professional mileage on them
to become skilled in helping the cerebral palsied individual manage
his unique problems. Beginning therapists are likely to approach their
first patients well informed about statistics relating to cerebral palsy
and with a list of techniques which they hope will work with their
patients. Unfortunately, patients can't be rehabilitated by statistics,
nor will they all respond favorably to the same treatment.

The reader will find that, instead of emphasizing the "facts and
figures" of cerebral palsy, this book concentrates on the "people" of
cerebral palsy—the children, their parents, and the professional workers.
Instead of presenting a method for treating cerebral palsied children,
this book introduces many of the methods which are used by various
professional groups and seeks principles which will guide the therapist
in employing these methods. The student who adds to the information
presented in this book the points of view of authors to which his attention is directed in the search items will have a sound foundation for
developing his clinical skills.

One cannot learn all he needs to know about the evaluation and
treatment of cerebral palsy from books or teachers. There is no substi-

tute for experience in working with patients. Unless however, the therapist has acquired basic information about cerebral palsy, contacts with patients are usually meaningless. The problems of cerebral palsied children are complex and difficult to solve. The cerebral palsied child has a right to expect that his therapists, though inexperienced, will be well informed.

E.T.M.

B.C.

contents

IT IS NOT TO BE EXPECTED THAT A TEXTBOOK WILL HAVE A CAST OF characters. In a very real sense this one does. The cast includes the person who is cerebral palsied, his parents and other members of his family, and the professional people who attempt to be of service to him and his family. In addition, there are many who play bit parts. These include neighbors, relatives, and friends. There are also many extras. Some of these merely stare at the cerebral palsied person in the street, but others give their time and money to support programs in which he is treated and educated. This is a large cast, but every one of the characters has some influence on the life of the person who is cerebral palsied. As we shall see, children with cerebral palsy are not habilitated by a doctor or a therapist. Rather, whatever degree of habilitation they achieve is the result of the cooperative effort of many people.

1 *cerebral palsy: the problems*

The various speech, physical, and occupational therapists play an important role in this drama of habilitation, but their's is not always the most important role. Without an understanding of the part to be played by all of the other members of this large cast, the therapists' act will fail to deserve much applause. A major purpose of this book is to help the therapist prepare to serve as an effective member of the professional group concerned with habilitating cerebral palsied individuals by:

1. Developing an understanding of the causes of cerebral palsy and a familiarity with the characteristics of the various types of cerebral palsy.
2. Developing an awareness of the various services essential to an adequate habilitation program for the cerebral palsied.
3. Developing an appreciation of the contributions made by various professional and lay groups involved in the habilitation process.
4. Development of a philosophy of rehabilitation which provides a basis for planning and action.

No one knows exactly how many persons there are in the United States who are cerebral palsied, but their number has been estimated at 550,000—a national agency estimates that every 53 minutes a new cerebral palsied child is born. The prevalence rate is estimated at about three per thousand population. Of the half million or so cerebral palsied persons in the United States, about one-third are under twenty-one years of age and two-thirds are over twenty-one years of age. In a New York State survey, six babies in every thousand live births were found to be cerebral palsied. The interested reader can find many more statistics about cerebral palsy. There are estimates of the number who are intellectually impaired, the number with defective speech, the number who have seizures; in fact, one can find a statistic pertaining to almost any aspect of cerebral palsy. Information of this type is valuable in understanding the broad features of the cerebral palsy problem and for developing effective programs for the cerebral palsied. Statistics, however, are cold and impersonal, and therapists

1   Compile tables of pertinent statistics relating to various aspects of cere-
     bral palsy such as incidence, types, mental ability, sensory impairments,
     etc. See (162), (174), also Altman (3: 4, 25), Ingram (90: 244), Cruick-
     shank (32), and Cardwell (20).

and teachers of cerebral palsied individuals are more interested in the individuals themselves than in the statistics about them. The following are some brief descriptions of the problems of a few cerebral palsied individuals who are part of the large group of a half million. The names used are fictitious, of course, but fictitious names are preferable to case numbers or initials because they help the student begin to think of persons rather than of diagnoses. The cases have been arranged to help the student get a little feeling for the significance of historical information, clinical observations, and test data. In each description sufficient information is provided to enable the reader to determine, or to develop an impression concerning, the type of cerebral palsy, the topography and severity of involvement, the possible etiology, the hearing, vision, speech, and language, the intelligence, the seizure status, the parent attitudes, and other factors important for programming habilitation. It is suggested that as the student works through those sections of this book dealing with classification, etiology, and associated problems, he reread these descriptions and work out a diagnosis and evaluation for each child.

Charles Pounka is eight years old. A full-term baby, he was cyanotic at birth and resuscitation measures were necessary. He appeared to be in good health when taken home from the hospital. Charles learned to roll over and sit in his crib, but his parents became suspicious that something was wrong when they noticed that he did not suck his thumb or learn to hold his bottle. Their suspicions grew stronger when Mr. Pounka realized that Charles used his feet rather than his hands to play with toys. Charles began walking at about fifteen months and at eight years of age his ambulation is satisfactory.

His parents noticed that Charles could recognize himself in the mirror when he was two years of age; also at that time he attempted to name many common objects, although his speech was not clear enough to understand. At four years of age, Charles was evaluated at a treatment center and the psychologist noted that Charles could indicate, by nodding his head, the correct answers to such questions as: Are you a girl? Is it morning now? Have you any brothers? He was unable to hold a pencil or crayon in his hand and he could not feed himself nor remove any of his clothing. It was often difficult for him to speak and his speech was usually intelligible only to persons who were familiar with him.

Charles began receiving speech therapy and occupational therapy at four years of age and entered a special school for handicapped children at seven years of age. At eight he has learned to read but can't write with the pencil held in his hand. His head and arms show a characteristic pattern—one arm is extended behind while the other is flexed in front of him. His head is rotated toward the extended arm. He easily brings his eyes to focus on objects. He is unable to feed himself because his mouth and arm are never in the same place at the same time. He can write and draw with a pencil held by the toes of his right foot. His parents and older brother are embarrassed to see Charles use his feet instead of his hands. His parents are worried about how anyone can learn to live independently if he can't use his hands. Mr. Pounka says he can't feed Charles any more because he can't stand to think that his son will "always eat like a baby."

Let us now present another cerebral palsied child. Four-year-old Clayton Penths, who weighed almost nine pounds at birth, is the third of four children. His siblings are all normal. Clayton rolls over with difficulty and cannot sit without support. When held in an upright position, he stands on his toes and his left leg crosses over in front of the right leg. He is unable to make any walking movements. Clayton is not yet toilet trained and his mother reports difficulty in spreading his legs apart for diapering him. His left eye is constantly turned in toward his nose. Until recently, Clayton had several seizures each day during which his eyes rolled upward, his arms and legs shook violently, and he made moaning sounds. Since he began receiving medication, the seizures occur only once or twice a month. Clayton can't hold toys or his bottle. It is difficult for his mother to feed him because he loses milk and baby foods from his mouth. He shows no sign of recognizing himself in a mirror. His vocalizations consist of vowel-like sounds with only an occasional consonant. These vocalizations occur in response to his mother's playing with him. He does not respond in any way to questions such as: Where is Daddy? Where is Mommy? Where is the light? Clayton responds to his mother's voice by smiling or turning his head. He is startled by the ringing of the phone or the doorbell. Mr. and Mrs. Penths are eager to schedule speech therapy and say they think Clayton will "come along all right once he learns to talk."

Another child, Charleen Pimskon, now three years of age, weighed about three pounds at birth. Charleen is an only child, but her mother had three pregnancies which terminated prematurely in stillbirths. Mr. and Mrs. Pimskon noticed that Charleen didn't kick much and that she was slow in learning to roll over, sit up, and crawl, but they attributed her slowness to her prematurity. Her mother noted on diapering Charleen that her legs appeared to be stiff and hard to move. Charleen began saying "mommy" and "daddy" at about one year and now, at three years of age, she uses sentences to carry on simple conversations. She can name most common objects correctly, count to five, and can repeat without error six-word sentences. Her speech is easy to understand. Charleen likes to listen to the record player and has learned to sing several nursery rhymes. Charleen seems to see satisfactorily, although first one eye and then the other turns outward away from the nose. When seated at a low table, she enjoys scribbling with a pencil and can cut paper with blunt scissors. She likes to play with blocks, can make a three-block pyramid, and can build a tower of eight blocks before they spill over. Charleen is unable to walk; when she is held in a standing position, she tends to stand on her toes while a scissoring of her legs occurs. A quick dorsiflexion of either foot causes the foot to continue jerking up and down until it is restrained. Mrs. Pimskon is angry with her family doctor who said that all prematures are slow and reassured her that Charleen would "come along O.K." She is also hurt by her mother-in-law who feels that something must be wrong with her since she loses so many babies. Mrs. Pimskon suspects that her husband holds some of the same feelings as his mother.

Catherine Pombst weighed only two pounds twelve ounces when she was born and was immediately placed in an isolette. Her parents were eager to bring her home from the hospital and when she was finally allowed to go home, they played with her a great deal. They noticed that Catherine did not follow them with her eyes, and when she was about a year of age, they began to suspect that she did not see. They also noticed that she had difficulty in learning to roll and sit. At about one year of age, however, Catherine began to say words, and by two, she could talk in short sentences and could eat with a spoon and drink from a cup without assistance. When Catherine was three years old, her difficulty was diagnosed as cerebral palsy with blindness, and physical therapy was initiated. She entered a residential school for cerebral palsied children when she was four years of age. Now at twelve years of age, Catherine reads Braille and is ambulatory with Canadian crutches. Catherine is becoming aware now that she is not like other children. She cries readily and has sudden flares of emotion and spells of moodiness. Her parents are very much concerned about her future. They realize that she will never get married and feel that she will probably never be able to live independently. Repeatedly they ask each other, "Who would take care of Catherine if anything happened to the two of us?"

Carl Pednok, now eight years old, was the pride and joy of his father. Carl said words at one year and was speaking in sentences at eighteen months. At four years of age, he could print his name, name common colors, and assemble simple jigsaw puzzles. He had been riding a tricycle since he was three. Carl loved to cut and paste and to have his older sister read to him. Shortly after his fourth birthday, Carl coasted down the family driveway on his tricycle and into the path of a truck which could not stop in time to avoid hitting him. Carl suffered a skull fracture and for several weeks after the accident he was unable to walk or talk. Gradually he learned to talk again, but he still misarticulates some sounds and he seems to have difficulty remembering the names of things. His right heel cord is tight, causing him to walk on the toes of his right foot; in walking he seems to use a trunk movement to throw his right leg around. The flexed right arm is held close to his body and his hand is tightly closed. When his eyes are shut he is unable to identify objects placed in his right hand, but he can readily identify the same objects when placed in his left hand. He uses his left hand for everything. For several months following his accident, Carl had spells during which he would lose consciousness and topple over. These spells occur now only if his mother forgets to give him his medicine. Carl attends a regular school but is having difficulty with reading. His teacher says he can't match forms and that he is easily distracted. At times Carl is quite aggressive with the other children. Carl's sister blames herself for his accident because she was supposed to be watching him. His father thinks Carl's mother was to blame. Mrs. Pednok thinks the teacher doesn't know how to manage Carl in school and thinks a better teacher could teach Carl to read.

Shortly after birth Clifford Puzin developed a yellow discoloration of the skin which cleared up after several days. He was a listless baby and had difficulty sucking and swallowing. His parents noted that Clifford did not cry or vocalize as much as his sister did when she was a baby. His parents thought he must be getting stronger because they noticed that he was frequently arching his back, touching the bed only with his heels and the back of his head. At two, however, he could not hold up his head or sit; at about that time, Clifford's parents learned that he was cerebral palsied. An evaluation when Clifford was four years old also revealed that he had a high-frequency hearing loss. He had little speech which could be understood and oftentimes it appeared that Clifford was trying to say something but couldn't make a sound. Psychological evaluation at this time was difficult because of his inability to use his hands and the unintelligibility of his speech. The psychologist noted that Clifford could nod appropriate answers to such questions as: Are you a boy? Are you a girl? Is it summer? Is it winter? Do you sleep on a table? Do you have a brother? You are six years old, aren't you?

When four colored squares were placed before him, he could look at the red one, the green one, the yellow one, or the blue one as directed. When four groups of blocks were placed before him, he could look at the group containing four blocks, three blocks, two blocks, or one block, as requested. Clifford entered a residential school for cerebral palsied children at five years of age for speech, physical and occupational therapy, and a special education program. Despite the use of a hearing aid and years of intensive speech and hearing therapy, Clifford's speech is still, at eighteen years of age, difficult to understand. Efforts to talk are accompanied by facial grimacing and drooling. He has learned to read well but cannot hold a book nor turn the pages. He can get around by himself, but his gait is awkward and unsteady. Clifford and his parents realize that it will be difficult for him to find employment in a competitive situation. They are wondering if he should enroll in a college or enter a sheltered workshop program. At times Clifford feels very depressed because he can't dance or talk with girls. His parents always feel uncomfortable when he wants to talk with them about such problems.

THE MEANING OF THE TERM "CEREBRAL PALSY"

The persons we have just described have in common the condition which today is generally called *cerebral palsy*. Their condition has not always been so named. In fact, the condition existed unnamed for many years. In the sculptured monuments of Egypt there are figures of individuals who appear to be cerebral palsied. In the Holy Scriptures there are many references to crippled individuals, some of whom appear to be cerebral palsied. Many early medical works contain references to the paralyses and deformities of crippled children. Early in the nineteenth century, physicians began to suspect that some of the crippling conditions were caused by brain lesions. One of the earliest clinical descriptions of a child who would today be considered cerebral palsied was made about the middle of the nineteenth century by an English surgeon, John Little. For many years thereafter the condition

2   What type of cerebral palsy did Dr. Little describe? Early in his professional life a student should begin reading primary sources. Wouldn't it be interesting to read what Dr. Little said (107: 378-80) before reading what Courville (28), Denhoff (43), and Cardwell (20) say he said?

was known as *Little's Disease.* Another commonly used label was *spastic.* These names tended to make people think that all cerebral palsied individuals were the same. As the six cases just described illustrate, this is far from being true. As diagnostic and evaluation procedures improved, marked variations in symptomatology were observed. Credit for coining the term *cerebral palsy* is given to Phelps. As used in the term, the word *cerebral* refers to the brain and the word *palsy* describes a lack of muscle control. Cerebral palsy is not a disease. Rather, as Perlstein (*137:* 47-52, 76) suggests, cerebral palsy is a term used to designate any paralysis, weakness, incoordination, or functional aberration of the motor system resulting from brain pathology. Lesions in different parts of the brain produce different symptoms of motor disfunction. Five common types of cerebral palsy have been identified: spastic, athetoid, rigidity, ataxic, and tremor. In addition, many subtypes, especially of the athetoids, have been described.

Not only do cerebral palsied children have motor problems, but often the brain lesion results in associated difficulties. It is not uncommon for cerebral palsied children to have one or more of the following: impaired vision, defective hearing, retarded intellectual development, defective speech, convulsions, orthopedic defects, dental anomalies, perceptual difficulties, and emotional problems. The cerebral palsied child might have in addition to his cerebral palsy any handicap that any child might have. In fact, he is more likely to have more of certain types of handicaps than are other children. Most cerebral palsied children are multiply handicapped. Not all, however, are severely handicapped. Some are so mildly involved that they are unnoticed and do not require any special attention. At the other extreme are many who are so severely involved that they will never learn to care for themselves. Fortunately, a large number of cerebral palsied persons whose early outlook seemed hopeless can, through appropriate treatment and education, be prepared for useful and satisfying places in society.

> 3   What skills and attitudes must adults possess in order for them to live happily and usefully in today's society, Analyze your own life and observe your associates. See Doll (46). Wright (193). Make a list of those skills and attributes which would be difficult for a severely involved cerebral palsied child to develop.

MULTIDISCIPLINARY AND COMPREHENSIVE PROGRAMS

Since most cerebral palsied children have one or more associated problems in addition to their primary motor disorder, it should be obvious that specialists representing numerous disciplines will be involved in the evaluation and management of the cerebral palsied child. During the 1950's there developed a considerable emphasis on what has been called the *team approach* to the management of cerebral palsied individuals. There is no standard pattern by which the various professionally trained individuals operate in evaluating and treating cerebral palsied persons. In some situations the team is highly organized. In other situations no "team" is officially organized, yet a group of professionally trained workers cooperate in applying their knowledge and skills to the problems of the cerebral palsied individual and his family. Obviously, no one individual, regardless of how highly trained, can possess all the knowledge and skills required for diagnosing and habilitating a cerebral palsied individual. In every instance, whether it regards itself as a "team" or not, a *group* of persons must be involved in the program of the cerebral palsied person.

Rembolt (*34*) says that a team approach is characterized by "concatenation" which he defines as "a series of links united; a series or order of things depending on each other as if linked; a chain." Rembolt suggests that the team approach, when viewed in this way, means "that all members of the team have some common objectives regarding the patient, that each member feels a certain amount of interdependence on his fellow team members, and that his interests in the patient are actively greater than those with which his specific field of specialization might have major concern." Whether a professional worker functions as a member of a highly organized team or as one of a loosely organized group, his perspective must extend beyond the boundaries of his own specialty. Effective habilitation of the cerebral palsied cannot be achieved by piecing together the efforts of many independently operating professional workers. Physicians, therapists, psychologists, educators, and everyone else concerned with the habilitation of cerebral palsied individuals must develop an awareness of the broad scope of the cerebral palsied individual's problems. They must become aware of all the needs of each cerebral palsied individual whom they serve; how their individual professional skills can best be employed to meet these needs; what contributions other professional and lay workers can make toward meeting these needs.

Regardless of how a team or group is organized, effective communication between its members is essential. There must be a pooling of information obtained from many specialities in order to arrive at an accurate evaluation of the cerebral palsied individual's problems. Pooling can take place only if the professional workers communicate with each other about their findings. Treatment, education, recreation, counseling, employment—all services—must be based on a knowledge of the total program plans for the cerebral palsied individual. Only through careful continuous coordination of their efforts can the various professional workers direct their services toward common objectives. Cerebral palsied individuals need a well planned *program* rather than merely a series of treatments.

SCOPE OF A COMPREHENSIVE PROGRAM

Recognizing that each of the half million cerebral palsied persons in the United States will have individual problems and that his problems and needs will change many times between birth and adulthood, professional and lay workers concerned with habilitating the cerebral palsied have often asked, "What are the essential features of a program which would most adequately meet the changing needs of cerebral palsied individuals?"

4   What disciplines would be represented on a team which is organized to habilitate cerebral palsied children and what services would a comprehensive rehabilitation program include? See Hanna (75: 5-8, 23), Denhoff (43), and (162).

In 1962, the Pennsylvania Society for Crippled Children and Adults, Inc., developed through a self-study the following description of a comprehensive rehabilitation program. The program is based on the recognition that individuals with handicaps, like all other persons, desire and have a right to live in dignity within the limits of their capabilities and to be responsible for their own welfare and destiny. The various aspects of the suggested program were derived from the belief that all persons with handicaps regardless of age, race, creed, color, type of handicap, financial status, or place of residence are entitled to the services needed for maximum development of their potential as accepted and contributing members of society. Further, the comprehensive program described recognizes that because problems of handicapped persons are shared by and contribute to those of their family members, programs and services for crippled children and adults must be family oriented rather than just patient oriented.

> 5   Work out a statement of the philosophy of rehabilitation which will guide you as you begin treating handicapped persons. Obtain from their national offices the policy statements of the National Society for Crippled Children, United Cerebral Palsy, The National Association for Retarded Children, and the U. S. Office of Vocational Rehabilitation. See also McDonald (108).

The large group of professional and lay persons involved in the Pennsylvania Society's self-study concluded that the scope of a comprehensive program of rehabilitation should be determined by the needs of the handicapped persons to be served rather than by the needs of professional and volunteer workers who serve them or the unpredictable urges of citizens who assist their handicapped brethren. While the following program outline was intended for individuals with all types of handicaps, it is especially appropriate for the cerebral palsied. A comprehensive program would include such features as:

1. *Prevention*—utilization of known procedures for preventing accidents and diseases which cause handicapping conditions.
2. *Case Finding*—the early identification of persons needing special attention because of a handicapping condition.
3. *Diagnosis and Evaluation*—provision of all the diagnostic and evaluative studies necessary for an adequate understanding of the nature of the handicapping condition and for the development of a plan for its management.
4. *Treatment*—all of the therapeutic procedures indicated by the diagnostic and evaluative studies.
5. *Education*
   a. educational programs appropriate to the needs and abilities of the handicapped person.
   b. education of the public concerning problems, needs, and potentials of handicapped persons and acceptance of them as full members of society.

6. *Counseling*—continuing psychological counseling for the handicapped person and his family.

7. *Employment*—vocational guidance, training, and job-placement services including sheltered-workshop programs for those unable to qualify for competitive employment.

8. *Recreation*—year-round recreational programs appropriate for handicapped persons of all ages who cannot participate in the normal leisure-time activities of their communities, and for the families of the handicapped, to provide an occasional release from their day-to-day responsibilities.

9. *Research*—support of research which may lead to a better understanding of the nature, causes, prevention, and treatment of handicapping conditions.

10. *Residential Care*—residential, institutional, and/or foster facilities appropriately designed and operated for the continuing care of severely handicapped persons who cannot live independently and whose care creates serious problems for their families.

11. *Financial Aid*—financial assistance, based upon need, for families who cannot afford the high cost of maintenance, support, and rehabilitation of a handicapped family member.

12. *Personnel Training*—recruitment and training of the professional, student, and volunteer lay personnel needed in all areas of a comprehensive program.

13. *Funding*—provision of funds through taxes or voluntary contribution to provide adequate financial support for the comprehensive program needed by handicapped persons and their families.

> 6   What organizations, voluntary and tax supported, in the United States are concerned with problems of cerebral palsy? See Messner's section in Illingworth (89).

To some readers this proposed rehabilitation program will appear to be an unattainable ideal. However, if we take as the basis of our programming the needs of cerebral palsied individuals, we cannot justify the elimination of any one of the thirteen aspects from our program. Partial programs may satisfy the need of the citizens to "do good" long before the needs of cerebral palsied persons are met. A program which recognizes only a few of his needs will not prepare the person with cerebral palsy "to live in dignity within the limits of his capabilities and to be responsible for his own welfare and destiny."

"WHAT CAUSED IT?" IS THE ANGUISHED QUESTION OF EVERY PARENT OF a cerebral palsied child. When told that cerebral palsy is a disorder of neuromuscular function due to malfunction of the brain, parents ask, "What's wrong in a child's brain when he has trouble in walking or talking or in using his hands?" Researchers and clinicians are also vitally interested in these questions. Complete answers are not available, but some understanding of the problems may be gained by studying the structure of the nervous system and its organization for sensory-motor function.

STRUCTURE OF THE NERVOUS SYSTEM

The nervous system consists of the brain, spinal cord, and peripheral

2 neurophysiologic bases and etiology of cerebral palsy

nerves. It is helpful in learning to understand the organization of the brain to begin with the three simple divisions which appear in an early differentiation of the neural tube during the embryonic stage of the organism. These divisions are the forebrain, the midbrain, and the hindbrain. By tracing the embryologic development of the brain, neuroanatomists have found that the forebrain divides into the *telencephalon,* or "endbrain," and the *diencephalon,* or "throughbrain." The midbrain, which does not subdivide, is sometimes called the *mesencephalon* which means "middle brain." The hindbrain divides into the *metencephalon,* or "afterbrain," and the *myelencephalon* which means "marrow brain."

7   The early bird isn't getting all the worms. Scientists are grabbing up some, training them, and then feeding the educated worms to uneducated cannibal worms. What happens then and what are the implications for our understanding of brain function? We'd like to tell you, but we have only 50,000 words to describe the foundations of cerebral palsy. Do you know what a neuron is and how a nerve impulse is transmitted? What happens at a synapse? What do you know about the function of the basal ganglia and what is the significance of recent investigations of the reticular formation and the gamma system? You will be a more effective member of a cerebral palsy rehabilitation group if you know more about the structure and function of the nervous system. For an easy start, read

"That Wonderful Machine, the Brain," *Fortune*, February 1963, pp. 125-29 and 184-92. Next, read Grayson's *Nerves, Brain and Man (71)*, and then get acquainted with an elementary text in neurology such as Gardner's *Fundamentals of Neurology (61)*. With this foundation you will be ready for Sherrington *(164)*, Penfield *(134)*, *(136)*, Granit *(69)*, Magoun *(111)*, and others.

The following outline shows how the several parts of the mature brain evolve from the embryonic neural tube.

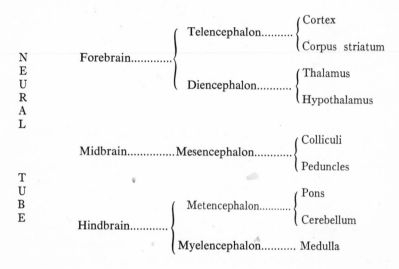

The cerebrum, which forms from the forebrain, is divided by a deep longitudinal fissure into the right and left cerebral hemispheres. The cortex, or outer layer, is composed of nerve cells and the interior is composed of nerve fibers. The major divisions of the brain are illustrated in Fig. 1.

Four systems of nerve fibers may be found in the cerebrum. The thalamocortical tracts link the cortex with the thalamus. Association tracts connect sensory areas with surrounding zones in the same hemisphere. Commissural tracts (called the *corpus callosum*) connect the two hemispheres. Projection fibers connect the cerebral hemispheres with lower parts of the nervous system.

8   When discussing the location of cortical lesions researchers and clinicians have used both functional classifications and the cytoarchitectural classifications of Brodmann. What are the bases for each of these methods of classification and into what areas does each divide the cortex? See CIBA Medical Illustrations *(125)*, von Bonin *(182)*, and Fulton *(60)*.

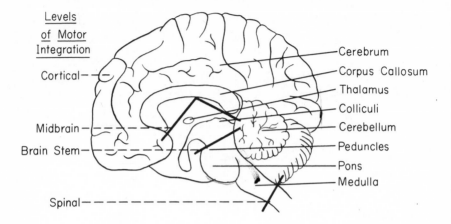

Figure 1. Medial View of Right Hemisphere and Sagittal Section of Brain, showing Major Divisions and Levels of Neural Integration of Motor Functions.

Pyramidal System

Fiber tracts descend without interruption from cell bodies in the fifth layer of the cortex to the level of the spinal cord where they synapse with the peripheral nerve that is also the final common path to the muscle innervated by the part of the cortex where the fiber originated. In the medulla about 80 per cent of the fibers cross to the opposite side before they descend in the cord. Hence, the left side of the body is controlled by the right side of the brain and vice versa. See Fig. 2 which illustrates the pyramidal tracts and the body representation in the motor cortex.

Extrapyramidal System

All fibers which are not included in the pyramidal tracts, but which can send impulses to the spinal cord from the brain, are regarded as part of the extrapyramidal system. In Fig. 3 it will be noted that these fibers do not descend without interruption from the cortex to the spinal cord. Rather, there are many connections with nuclei in the thalamus, the basal ganglia, the midbrain, the cerebellum, the medulla, and the reticular formation.

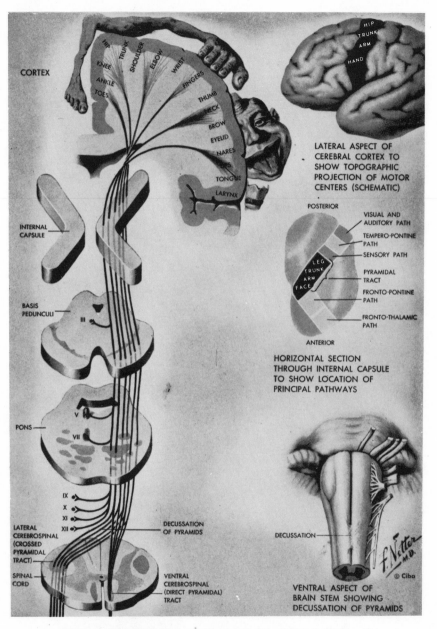

Figure 2. Pyramidal System. (Copyright *The CIBA Collection of Medical Illustrations*, by Frank H. Netter, M.D.)

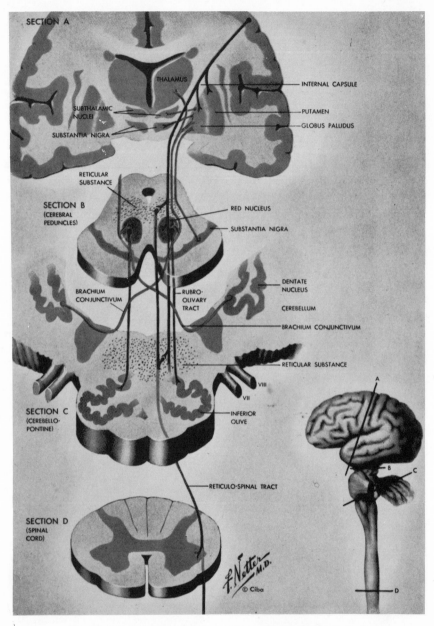

SECTION A

THALAMUS
INTERNAL CAPSULE
SUBTHALAMIC NUCLEI
PUTAMEN
GLOBUS PALLIDUS
SUBSTANTIA NIGRA

RETICULAR SUBSTANCE

SECTION B
(CEREBRAL PEDUNCLES)
RED NUCLEUS
SUBSTANTIA NIGRA

BRACHIUM CONJUNCTIVUM
RUBRO-OLIVARY TRACT
DENTATE NUCLEUS
CEREBELLUM
BRACHIUM CONJUNCTIVUM

RETICULAR SUBSTANCE
VIII
VII
SECTION C
(CEREBELLO-PONTINE)
INFERIOR OLIVE

RETICULO-SPINAL TRACT

SECTION D
(SPINAL CORD)

F. Netter, M.D.
© Ciba

A
B
C

D

Figure 3. Extrapyramidal System. (Copyright *The CIBA Collection of Medical Illustrations*, by Frank H. Netter, M.D.)

ORGANIZATION FOR SENSORY-MOTOR FUNCTION

Muscular activity is involved in every motor act. Muscles act in response to stimuli from the nervous system, hence, for every motor reaction there must be an adequate stimulus. Sensory receptors do not have direct neural connections with muscles. Before a sensory stimulus can activate a muscle, an afferent stimulus must be sent from the sensory receptor to the central nervous system from which an efferent stimulus will be transmitted to a selected muscle as illustrated in Fig. 4.

Sensations may arise from external stimuli or from within the body itself. Sensitive exteroceptors are responsive to many types of environmental conditions and signal needs for motor action to the central nervous system. Proprioceptive sensations are especially important for control of motor activity.

9   Proprioception is now regarded as one of the most highly developed senses. Cerebral palsy specialists have related some of the motor problems of the cerebral palsied child to his patterns of proprioceptive sensation, and techniques for modifying proprioceptive stimulation are employed in some therapies. What are the proprioceptive receptors and how does proprioception effect muscle function? See Gardner (61), Sherrington (164), Granit (69), Hellebrandt (81: 9-14).

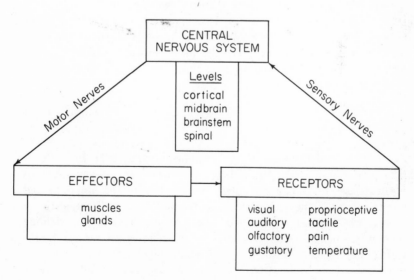

Figure 4. Reaction Mechanism for Sensory-Motor Function.

Motor mechanisms normally operate under the control of several levels of the central nervous system. This does not mean that each part of the nervous system can function independently. The nervous system as a whole contributes to each motor act with the higher levels dominating the lower levels.

Spinal Level

The lowest level of motor integration takes place in the spinal cord. Homolateral or contralateral reflexes occur when afferent impulses enter a segment of the cord and stimulate a motor neuron exiting from that segment to a muscle on the same side or to a muscle on the opposite side. Longitudinal spinal reflexes occur when afferent impulses travel to higher or lower levels of the cord before synapsing with a motor neuron. Three reflexes associated with movements of the limbs are mediated at this level: the flexor withdrawal reflex, the extensor thrust, and the cross extensor reflex. In normal development these reflexes come under the control of higher centers, but this higher level control does not develop in some cerebral palsied children.

Pontine Level

At this level, which is also called the *brain-stem level,* afferents from receptors in the labyrinths of the ear and from the muscles of the neck enter the central nervous system. Head positions give rise to afferent stimuli which synapse with motor neurons in the brain stem to produce postural reactions. For example, the asymmetrical tonic neck reflex seen in normal infants and in many older cerebral palsied children is mediated at this level.

Midbrain Level

Reflexes at the spinal level are responses to stimulation applied to narrowly limited body areas. For example, if you strike the patellar tendon, the knee jerks. At the brain-stem level reflexes and reactions are responses to stimuli generated by receptors in the labyrinth and proprioceptors in the neck muscles. At the midbrain level tactile stimuli arising from the body surface modify motor responses. Several righting reflexes are integrated at this level. These reflexes are related to the child's development through predictable stages of motor function progressing from rolling over to standing. In normal children these reflexes gradually come under the inhibition of cortical control. Cerebral palsied children often have difficulty developing these important patterns of motor function.

Cortical Level

At this level the nervous system has access to stimuli from all the body's receptors. The intact and mature nervous system operating at this level has control of its motor activities and can modify them as needed to meet environmental conditions.

> **10** All types of cerebral palsy are characterized by abnormalities of movement resulting from maldevelopment of, or injury to, the brain. How does the normal central nervous system organize patterns of movement? See Wenger (*183*), Magoun (*111*), Denny-Brown (*44*), Penfield (*136*).

DEFECTIVE ORGANIZATION FOR SENSORY-MOTOR FUNCTION

Damage to, or maldevelopment of, some part of the brain prevents the normal development of the integrative processes which are basic to normal motor functioning. Lower levels of the central nervous system operate without the control of higher levels. Tonic reflex patterns, tremors, and other uncontrolled motor mechanisms interfere with the development of normal sequences of motor activities. Several groups of symptoms of motor malfunctioning—spasticity, athetosis, tremors, rigidity, ataxia—result from the brain lesion. The symptoms present depend in part on where in the brain the lesion is located.

ETIOLOGY

Parents, researchers, and clinicians want to know what causes the brain lesions which result in cerebral palsy? The answer will be found in a study of those conditions which interfere with the development of the brain or which result in damage to a normally developing brain. The conditions which produce symptoms of cerebral palsy might occur before birth, during birth, immediately following birth, or even later. See Perlstein (*137*: 47-52, 76), Deaver (*36*: 532-36), Greenspan (*72*: 478-85), Keith (*94*: 190-204), Evans (*51*: 213-19).

Prenatal Factors

Prenatal factors may be either congenital or acquired. Congenital factors are those which are transmitted through the genes; thus from the time of conception they are present to interfere with fetal development. Acquired factors are those intrauterine conditions which are hostile to the unborn infant.

Human beings begin their embryonic development as a speck of living matter which even under a microscope shows no resemblance to human features.[1] By the time he is ready for delivery into the outer world, the human infant has developed from his original one cell into an organism of over a trillion cells. In this development some cells form muscles and bones, whereas others differentiate to become organs; from a third group of cells, the brain, spinal cord, nerves, and sense organs emerge. During this developmental process, cells must grow, divide, and even migrate. They must interact with other tissues; they must develop differential and unique characteristics (133). All these processes are so fantastically complex and so many things can go wrong that we marvel that so many people are born to be normal.

There is a growing awareness that genetic factors are responsible not only for traits such as blue eyes or red hair, but also that defective genes may produce mental retardation, cerebral palsy, microcephaly, cleft palate, muscular dystrophy, and many other congenital malformations or malfunctions (58).

Genetic factors can also be responsible for blood incompatibilities as when the mother's blood is Rh negative and the child's blood is Rh positive. Metabolic disturbances such as diabetes sometimes have a genetic basis. Blood incompatability and maternal metabolic disturbances can lead to cerebral palsy in the child.

> 11   It has been estimated that at least 10 per cent of cerebral palsy cases have their origin in hereditary factors. By what mechanisms do genetic factors result in malformations and malfunctions? See Fishbein, ed (58), Dick and Stevenson (45: 921-23), Schut (160: 535-68), Powdermaker (148: 148), Ginsburg (67: 257).

The most common cause of acquired cerebral palsy during the prenatal stage is anoxia. A pregnant woman can encounter a number of conditions which could cause a reduction in the amount of oxygen in her blood. Probably the most common of these conditions is the coma following a severe accident. During the comatose state, the mother's

> [1]For a delightful and informative discussion of how man develops from that "unfelt, unknown, and unhonored instant when a minute, wriggling sperm plunges headlong into a mature ovum" until, nine months later, he enters the outer world as a "squalling, seven pound (more or less) baby," read Margaret Shea Gilbert's *Biography of the Unborn* (Baltimore: The Williams and Wilkins Company, 1938).

respiratory function is depressed: the oxygen level in her blood falls, and the fetus consequently suffers an oxygen deficit. Since the infant's blood is oxygenated through an exchange of oxygen and carbon dioxide across the placental barrier, placental bleeding, placenta praevia, or infarcts in the placenta would also interfere with the oxygen supply to the fetus. Sometimes the maternal circulation is normal and the placenta is intact, but the umbilical cord does not deliver an adequate oxygen supply to the fetus because of kinks or because the cord is compressed between the head of the fetus and the mother's pelvis.

Because they produce harmful alterations in the chemistry of the fetal environment, maternal infections (particularly those which occur during the first trimester of pregnancy) can lead to damage of the fetal brain. Viral infections, particularly rubella, sometimes lead to damage of brain cells. Overexposure to X rays, which might occur during an examination of a mother to determine the fetal position, may result in damaged brain tissue.

The prenatal period has appropriately been referred to as "the fateful months when life begins." It is estimated that the causes of 30 per cent of all cerebral palsy cases occur during these months.

Natal Factors

A human being's trip through the birth canal is probably the most hazardous journey any individual will ever make. Powerful contractions of uterine muscles force him from a lodging which will no longer tolerate him. His exodus is obstructed by the bony barrier of his mother's pelvic girdle. Since he must use his head to get into the outer world, it is fortunate that the bones of the skull are not rigidly joined together. This arrangement permits a certain amount of movement without fracturing the bones or damaging the underlying brain tissues. But there are times when this journey into the outside world cannot be made without obstetric assistance.

During his fetal period, the infant was well protected from bumps and jars by being encased in a fluid-filled sac. At an early stage of the birth process the amniotic sac ruptures and the infant must make his way through the narrow confines of the birth canal without his protective water jacket. Most infants make their way through the birth canal with nothing more than a bruise or two to show for their bumps. As soon as he emerges from the birth canal, the infant gasps for breath and then utters a cry. His parasitic existence is over. From this time on the child carries on his own biological functions.

However, many things may occur during delivery which can cause damage to the brain. Delivery which occurs too rapidly does not permit time for adjustments between the intrauterine pressure and the atmospheric pressure or for the proper molding of the head to fit the birth canal. Both of these failures can produce the escape of blood from the cerebral blood vessels and result in damage to brain tissue. During a prolonged delivery the baby's head may be pounded on the bony floor of the mother's pelvis causing excessive traumatization of the brain. Difficult births sometimes make it necessary for the obstetrician to manipulate the fetus or to apply forceps to the head to assist in the delivery. In either of these procedures, brain damage might occur. Even in a Cesarean delivery there are two factors which sometimes result in brain damage: (a) the rapid delivery does not allow for the gradual adjustment of the fetal circulatory system from the intrauterine condition to that of atmospheric pressure and (b) the Cesarean surgery interrupts the fetal-maternal circulatory system.

> 12   Therapists often take case histories from mothers whose children are not
>   developing normally. Make a list of those aspects of the birth history
>   which might be suggestive of brain damage. See Anderson (4: 3-8),
>   Denhoff (40).

Being born has been described as the most difficult time of a person's life. It is likely that a great many children suffer some slight injury to the cerebrovascular system during this time because red cells are frequently found in the cerebrospinal fluid after birth. Usually such damage is minimal and the child suffers no lasting effects from it. In other children the sequelae are severe enough to result in motor disabilities, emotional problems, mental retardation, language disturbances, or perceptual difficulties which interfere with learning.

Neonatal Period

The child's problems do not end with his delivery. He has to adjust to the marked differences between intrauterine and atmospheric pressures. No longer can his tissues get their oxygen supply from his mother through the placenta. He must learn to breathe for himself—and quickly, too, for his brain cannot function long without oxygen.

The period immediately following birth also has hazards. Anything which interferes with the establishment of the infant's respiratory function is a potential cause of cerebral palsy. Excessive use of medication to produce maternal anesthesia or analgesia during labor can conceivably result in a suppression of the infant's respiratory center.

If plugs of mucus are present in the infant's respiratory tract they obstruct the flow of air and prevent the lungs from expanding. If for any reason the child's breathing mechanism cannot provide an adequate supply of oxygen for his body tissues severe damage to brain tissues may occur.

The incidence of cerebral palsy is higher among premature infants than among those carried to full term. A premature baby is one weighing five and a half pounds or less at birth regardless of whether it is born at the normal nine-month period of gestation or before. Some premature babies are so poorly developed that they cannot be kept alive. Others, with proper care, will continue growing and will eventually complete the development of their underdeveloped parts and functions. The great majority of premature babies who survive infancy grow up into normal, healthy adults. But there are others who do not. Among the hazards which occasionally interfere with the normal development of "premies" are delicate blood vessels in the brain. These break easily and the resulting hemorrhage damages brain tissue.

Postnatal Factors

Brain damage can occur even to the child who has developed normally during the prenatal period, survived the hazards of birth, and run the gauntlet of the neonatal period. Accidents can still happen and diseases occur. Anything which adversely affects the brain after birth is a potential cause of cerebral palsy. Fractures of the skull or penetrating head wounds may result from accidents. Infections such as encephalitis and brain abscesses may occur during childhood as well as later in life. Cerebral hemorrhage might result from the rupture of a congenital aneurysm of a brain vessel. Poisoning such as lead encephalopathy is uncommon today, but it still remains a potential postnatal cause of cerebral palsy. Brain tumors, if permitted to expand, may damage brain cells as may the surgical removal of the neoplasm. Motor malfunction is a common sequelae of each of these cerebral pathologies.

Role of Anoxia and Hemorrhage

As we have seen, there are many possible causes of cerebral palsy. These causes usually damage the brain by producing anoxia which deprives the brain cells of needed oxygen or by causing a cerebral hemorrhage.

Brain cells are especially sensitive to oxygen deprivation. If they are without an adequate oxygen supply for even a few minutes, brain cells suffer irreparable damage. To provide the brain with oxygen and nutrients a rich blood supply is necessary; hence, the surface of the brain is almost covered with networks of blood vessels. Cerebral arteries send branches to all parts of the brain and venous sinuses are located strategically to drain blood from the brain. During the birth process the veins and sinuses on the surface of the brain are sometimes torn and cells in the cerebral cortex are damaged by the hemorrhaging. Abrupt pressure changes may cause rupturing of vessels in cortical and subcortical areas. Also, spasms may occur in arteries causing these vessels to rupture. Occasionally an artery will "blow out" because of a congenital weakness in the arterial wall. Anoxia may lead to hemorrhaging because an inadequate supply of oxygen makes blood-vessel walls more permeable and fragile.

13   Review the blood supply of the brain and determine what parts of the brain would be damaged by rupture of a meningeal blood vessel, superior sagittal sinus, or the lenticular striate artery. See *Nervous System,* Ciba Medical Illustrations *(125)* and Anderson *(41:* 3-8).

Brain cells also may be damaged by pressure from a tumor, by abnormal accumulation of cerebrospinal fluid within the skull, by such direct mechanical mutilation as penetration of a bullet[1] or bone fragment, or by toxic chemicals which change the molecular composition of the cell. The most common causes of brain-cell damage in infantile cerebral palsy, however, are anoxia and hemorrhage.

Lesions and Symptoms

Attempts have been made to correlate etiological factors with locations of lesions in the brain and with symptomatology. The skilled neurologist can determine with a high degree of precision the site of lesion which produces certain symptoms in an individual who had a fully developed central nervous system prior to the lesion. Such precision is not possible, however, when examining a child whose lesion occurred before patterns of central nervous system function had developed.

[1]We saw a cerebral palsied child whose psychotic father attempted to murder his family and then committed suicide by shooting himself. The child survived because the bullet missed a vital spot in his head, but he was cerebral palsied because of his brain damage.

Some of the published information concerning lesions in children's brains is based on post-mortem studies of children who have long been institutionalized. Institutionalized children tend to be very severely involved neurologically. Seldom are post-mortem studies done on the brains of mildly or moderately involved children. Much of our information is inference based on descriptions of symptoms resulting from certain lesions in adults. Animal experimentation has enabled researchers to develop much basic knowledge about the relationship of experimentally created lesions to behavioral change. But there are dangers in interpreting human behavior in terms of the results of animal experiments. The unique degree of telencephalization found in the organization of the human nervous system makes the function of the human brain significantly unlike the function of animal brains in many important respects.

One point of view holds that it is not possible to predict the nature, the exact location, or the degree of severity of the brain lesion on the basis of neurological symptoms. Another point of view suggests that the various types of cerebral palsy may be classified according to the anatomic site of the brain lesion. The following correlations between etiology, site of brain lesion, and symptoms have gained a rather wide acceptance among clinicians but are less well accepted by researchers in neuroanatomy and neurophysiology:

1. Pyramidal tract lesions, whether in the motor area of the cortex or in the area of the internal capsule are said to produce the symptoms of spasticity.
2. The patterns of involuntary movement seen in the athetoid and tremor types of cerebral palsy have been attributed to damage to the extrapyramidal system, especially to the nuclei of the basal ganglia.
3. Ataxia has been associated with cerebellar lesions.
4. Rigidity has been attributed to extrapyramidal involvement.
5. Anoxia is cited as a frequent cause of extrapyramidal lesions, while histories of hemorrhaging or trauma are associated with pyramidal tract symptoms.

> 14 While the clinician speaks of cerebral palsy in terms of pyramidal tract involvement and extrapyramidal tract involvement, neurophysiologists, on the basis of neuroanatomy, question the validity of distinguishing between the pyramidal and extrapyramidal systems. What other classical views of neuroanatomy and neurophysiology as related to cerebral palsy are being challenged today? See Courville in (34), Perlstein (138: 30-34), Meyers in (89).

Actually, while much has been written about the etiology of cerebral palsy, the nature and location of the lesions producing the various patterns of symptoms are not yet fully understood. There are several sources from which better information will be forthcoming. Through the Brain Registry of the American Academy for Cerebral Palsy, brains of deceased cerebral palsied children are sectioned and studied in order to determine the nature of the pathology which produced the child's cerebral palsy. Explorations of the living human brain made possible by advances in neurosurgical techniques are yielding much new information about the organization of the central nervous system. The National Institute of Neurological Diseases and Blindness together with fifteen medical centers are collaborating in studying approximately 50,000 pregnant mothers and their children in an attempt to determine the possible relationship between unfavorable factors present during pregnancy, labor, and early infancy and the neurological disorders which appear in the children.

> 15   What is the design of the Collaborative Perinatal Research Project and what potential etiological factors and possible sequelae of brain damage is it investigating? See (24) and (116).

Therapists will want to keep informed of new findings concerning etiology and the nature of the brain lesions which cause neurological deficits. These findings will undoubtedly have future implications for the development of therapeutic and educational measures. Fortunately for the cerebral palsied child, however, the therapist and teacher do not need accurate information about the cause of his cerebral palsy or the site of his lesion in order to be of assistance to him in learning to walk, talk, develop self-help skills and in learning to read and write.

Let us now return to the persons with cerebral palsy whom we met in Chapter I. From her history it appears that Catherine Pombst was a "premie" and suffered a hemorrhage which affected her control of both legs. What might have been the etiological factors in the cases of Charles Pounka, Clayton Penths, Charleen Pimskon, and Carl Pednok?

DIAGNOSIS IS THE PROCESS OF DETERMINING THE NATURE OF A disease or of a pathological condition. A diagnosis is determined by a review of the case history, an analysis of the symptoms described, and an interpretation of the signs or objective evidence of pathology. A differential diagnosis involves distinguishing one pathological condition from another. The diagnosis of cerebral palsy consists of determining if there is any alteration of neuromuscular function resulting from a brain lesion. This determination is made by a physician who studies the prenatal, natal, and postnatal history for factors which might have produced a maldeveloped or a damaged brain. He observes the child's motor behavior, watching for abnormalities of posture and movement, and, by examination, he attempts to elicit signs of lesions in the central nervous system. Not all children whose posture and movements are

3   *diagnosis and classification*

not normal for their age are cerebral palsied. Cerebral palsy must be differentiated from many other conditions such as peripheral nerve injuries, mental retardation, muscular dystrophy, infantile paralysis, vestibular dysfunction, and myasthenia gravis, to name a few.

> 16   Make a list of the conditions which interfere with normal neuromuscular development in children and show how cerebral palsy may be differentiated from these conditions. See Denhoff and Holden (42: 452-56), Illingworth (89), and Chusid and McDonald (23).

INITIAL MEDICAL EXAMINATION OF A CHILD SUSPECTED OF BEING CEREBRAL PALSIED

Beginning therapists watching a physician examine a child suspected of being cerebral palsied often feel in the dark about what the physician is doing. The following "play by play" description will help the therapist become a more intelligent observer and participant on clinic days.

The first objective of the physician is to determine whether or not something is wrong with the child's neuromuscular function. In a large percentage of cases it is possible for the physician to make this determination as soon as he sees the child. The physician's information gathering begins with the apparently casual observations he makes when the mother and child enter the examination situation. Since part of his early assessment will be based on comparing the child's developmental level with normal developmental patterns, the physician needs to know the age of the child he is examining. It is unsafe to estimate the child's age on the basis of his size because, not only do many cerebral palsied children develop motor skills more slowly, but they also tend to be physically smaller than normal children of the same age. The reaction of the child to his mother, the reactions of the mother

17 Compare the physical and motor development of cerebral palsied children with that of average children of the same age. See Ruby and Matheny (*153:* 525-27) and Denhoff and Holden (*42:* 452-56).

to the child, and the reactions of both to the clinic situation may provide important clues in diagnosing the child's problem.

Nonambulatory Child

The physician notes the posture of a nonambulatory child, paying attention to such items as head control, sitting balance, and trunk posture. The manner in which a child uses his upper extremities, his facial expressions, and his eye coordination might be indicative of some neuromuscular difficulties. By making these observations as the child is held in his mother's arms or sits in her lap, an experienced physician is often able to make a tentative diagnosis of the child's condition. Therapists might wonder what the physician saw in these few minutes to indicate a diagnosis of cerebral palsy. To the trained and experienced eye, lack of head control, evidenced by head dropping, is indicative of muscle weakness. Imbalance of eye muscles with resultant squint or abnormal motions is suggestive of spasticity. Sitting with rounded shoulders and with loss of normal lordosis of the lower back with the spine curved forward and prominent is indicative of neuromuscular malfunction. Sometimes the child will be observed to sit with the neck and spine in extension. Arms, when held in a flexed position or in extreme extension, are indications of neuromuscular difficulty. Sometimes a persistent asymmetrical tonic neck reflex or involuntary motions in the upper extremities will be seen. Careful observation of the hands may reveal fingers clenched with the thumb inside the palm, the so-called *cerebral thumb.*

In cerebral palsy the wrists may be flexed and deviated, usually to the ulnar side. Looking carefully at the legs, the physician may note

18   You will encounter many new words as you study and work in the field of cerebral palsy. To make your reading more meaningful, develop your own glossary and add new words regularly. Use sketches as well as verbal definitions in your glossary. Check several sources before writing your definitions. As a starter, what does ulnar mean?

that they are drawn up against the abdomen, or, if the child has an extensor pattern, the legs may be held in extreme extension and sometimes crossed. In a spastic child one foot or both feet might be in plantar flexion, that is, with the toes pointing toward the floor. The child's legs may be held in an extreme frog position, that is, flexed and abducted from the hip. Any of these conditions would be indicative of neuromuscular dysfunction.

Obviously an emotionally upset child who is crying and tense will not reveal a normal picture of his muscle function. For this reason, the physician tries to learn as much as possible from observing the child as he sits on his mother's lap rather than immediately undressing and beginning to manipulate the child. However, it is entirely possible that a cerebral palsied child who is physically and emotionally secure in his mother's arms will not show any abnormalities. Therefore, knowing that neurological abnormalities will be accentuated by reducing the child's security, the physician may next have the mother hold the child in a standing position with its feet on the floor. In this position any spasticity present will be increased and any abnormal motions will be emphasized. The physician also notes if the child needs the full support of his mother or if he can stand when held by only one hand. Also of interest is whether or not the child can take any steps with full or partial support.

After making these observations, the physician will have the mother return the child to her lap and remove his shoes and stockings to allow for the testing of reflexes and further observing of involuntary motions. The ankle jerk and knee jerk will be stimulated and observed for the hyperactivity characteristic of spasticity. Clonus in the calf muscle as manifested in repetitive flexion-extension of the foot will be noted. With the child still on his mother's lap the physician will test for increased reflexes at the elbow and wrist and will note changes in muscle tone. When testing a child suspected of being cerebral palsied, the physician may not test for pathological reflexes such as the Babinski. Pathologic reflexes are helpful in diagnosing acquired neurological lesions in adults, but they are not consistent in children who are brain damaged from birth.

> 19   While they are not all employed in studying cerebral palsied children, four types of reflexes are of importance in neurodiagnosis. Identify the four types and determine their diagnostic significance. Describe the stimulus and response for each of the following reflexes: biceps, triceps, patellar, Achilles, plantar, and Babinski. See Chusid and McDonald (23) and De Jong (39).

In examining small children the physician might again use the mother's lap as his examining table for the next part of his examination. While the child is lying on his back with his clothing removed, the physician will once more note muscle tone, presence of involuntary motion, and the range of motion in the joints of the upper and lower extremities. Particular attention will be given to the hip joints because muscular imbalance, particularly in spastics, often results in partial or total dislocation of the hip. Restricted range of motion is suggestive of neuromuscular malfunction and influences to some degree the type of physical therapy program recommended. Throughout his examination of the nonambulatory patient the physician is alert for signs of persistent primitive reflex patterns.

> 20   When evaluating and treating cerebral palsied children, some physicians and therapists are influenced by the presence of spinal, brain-stem, and midbrain reflex patterns. What are these reflexes and how are they elicited? See Chusid and McDonald (23), Mysak (122), and Bobath (15: 4-10).

The Ambulatory Child

With the ambulatory patient, just as with the nonambulatory patient, the physician begins his assessment as soon as the child enters the room. First he looks for deviations from the normal walking pattern. Simply stated, the elements of a normal walking pattern would be as follows: the individual stands upright with the head held erect and the shoulders back. Normal walking is characterized by a heel-toe gait in which the heel strikes first and the walker pushes off with the toes. The weight-bearing foot is planted firmly on the floor. A line projected downward from the anterior of the pelvis would fall through the knee-cap and strike the foot at the second toe. The weight-bearing knee is straight. The pelvis lifts when the non-weight-bearing leg is flexed. The walking movement occurs as a smooth, coordinated reciprocal pattern.

> 21   In the normal child, walking is achieved only after the child has passed through a number of stages during which he developed the neuro-

muscular prerequisite for walking. What are the physical achievements which a child must attain before he can walk? See Gesell (*63*), Shriner (*166*), and Shirley (*165*).

Deviations from this normal walking pattern make the physician suspect some neuromuscular dysfunction. The following observations are strongly suggestive of spasticity: a gait in which one leg crosses in front of the other due to tightness in the adductors and weakness in the abductors of the hip; walking with the knees bent due to slow contraction time in the quadriceps and tight hamstrings; forward flexion of the trunk due to an attempt to maintain balance and a weakness in the hip extensors. Walking on the toes with the heels off the ground results from spasticity in the calf muscles. Poor foot position suggests spasticity and/or imbalance in the invertors and evertors of the foot. In spasticity there is usually a flexor pattern in the upper extremities with the elbow and wrist being held in a flexed position. In hemiplegia these patterns would be observed on only one side.

A patient who walks like the spastic with his knees bent, but whose arms are in a position suggestive of a remnant of some early tonic reflex pattern, and whose patterns are variable is probably an athetoid. Facial grimaces during the walking makes the physician think of athetosis.

Some patients will be observed to shuffle along with a broad base, that is, with their feet far apart and not lifted far from the floor. Their knees will not be bent as are the spastic's. When one of these patients walks barefooted his toes are flared and act as if they are gripping the ground. Such a patient might be an ataxic. A severe ataxic might stagger from side to side and try to support himself by holding to the wall. He has a loss of position sense and may not know when he is falling.

Two other walking patterns might make the physician suspicious of cerebral palsy. If, when a child stands on one leg in order to lift the other one for taking a step, a tremor in the standing leg throws the child off his stride, the physician looks for other signs of tremor athetosis. Tremors in the lower extremities are likely to spread to other parts of the body. Yet another child may be observed to walk with the knees flexed but without the scissoring of the spastic. His motions are slow and deliberate and his walking pattern leads the physician to suspect rigidity.

After observing the gait of the child, either as he enters the examination room or walks in response to instructions, the physician would examine the child on a table to look for hyperactive reflexes, assess

muscle tone, and range of motion, and to look for signs of involuntary
motion.

> 22   Physical and occupational therapists and physicians frequently use terms
> such as the following to describe joint motions: flexion, extension, abduc-
> tion, adduction, pronation, supination, inversion, eversion, rotation, and
> opposition. Learn what each of these terms means and be able to demon-
> strate the motion at major joints. See Duvall (48).

A clinical evaluation of the type just described will usually enable
the physician to determine whether or not the child has cerebral palsy.
It will also provide him with enough information to specify the type
of cerebral palsy and the topography of involvement; in addition it
will permit him to make an estimate of the severity of the child's condition. If the professional group to be responsible for the child's program is oriented to thinking of treatment as an opportunity to learn
more about the nature of the child's problems, a clinical evaluation of
this type will yield enough information to get the child's program
under way. It must be remembered, however, that a cerebral palsied
child must visit a clinic many times before he becomes acclimated
sufficiently for the staff to see him "as he really is." This means that
program suggestions made after the initial examination should be regarded as tentative and intended primarily to give direction to activities
which will produce additional information about the child. Program
planning cannot be based solely on an initial diagnosis. Effective program plans must be developed through observations made during
treatment and a number of evaluations.

SPECIAL MEDICAL EXAMINATIONS

The neuromuscular problems of many cerebral palsied children will
be revealed by the clinical examination of a physician with special
training and experience in the diagnosis and treatment of cerebral
palsy. In any clinic, however, children will be seen whose problems
cannot be so readily diagnosed. These children do not show the typical
patterns of cerebral palsy. Some have enjoyed a period of normalcy
before their development was interrupted by a brain-tissue-destroying
condition such as infectious encephalitis, a brain trauma resulting from
an accident, or the surgical removal of a brain tumor. A relatively
small group of children who might be confused with the cerebral palsied
are those with hypotonic diseases of muscles such as amyotonia, congenital hypotonia (the child who is referred to as a *floppy baby*), and
myasthenia gravis.

The physician may in certain instances decide to supplement his clinical examination with certain special medical examinations. The following is a brief description of the special examinations which a physician is most likely to order for a cerebral palsied child.

Electroencephalogram

The electroencephalogram, commonly referred to as an *EEG*, is a record of electrical voltages or brain waves as picked up by miniature electrodes attached to several different regions of the scalp. The procedure, which is painless for the patient, produces information about the electrical activity of the brain. Electrical impulses picked up from the brain are amplified to many times their original strength. The amplified voltages operate pens which record on a moving tape the pattern of the brain's electrical activity. Normal brain waves recorded from all regions of the brain tend to be rhythmic. Abnormal rhythms are associated with brain pathology. By indicating the region in which the dysrhythmia occurs, electroencephalograms are helpful in determining the location of the pathological condition. An EEG might also reveal the presence of subclinical seizures which might interfere with learning and influence behavior without producing overt convulsions.

23 Make drawings to illustrate the EEG of a normal adult while awake, a normal adult while asleep, and an adult with a history of convulsions. How do they differ? See Hughes (85), Chusid and McDonald (23), Penfield (135).

Pneumoencephalogram

Within the brain are four cavities, the ventricles. These cavities communicate with each other, with a space between the arachnoid and pia mater (two of the membranous coverings of the brain and spinal cord), and with the central canal of the spinal cord. Cerebrospinal fluid circulates within the ventricles, central canal, and subarachnoid space to bathe the surfaces of the brain and the spinal cord. By inserting a needle into the spinal subarachnoid space while the child is under general anesthesia, a neurosurgeon can remove some of the cerebrospinal fluid and replace it with air. X-ray films are then made of the child's head. In the X-ray film the brain tissue and air have sufficient contrast to reveal the size and configuration of the ventricles and the appearance of the brain surface. The pneumoencephalogram is useful in revealing certain types of intracranial pathology such as cortical, cerebral, and cerebellar atrophy. The technique is not without risks and many children are ill for a few days afterward. Specialists do not agree about its usefulness for diagnosis and prognosis in cerebral palsy.

> 24   Where is the cerebrospinal fluid formed? What is the pattern of its
>   circulation? How is the quantity regulated? See Ciba (125), Chusid and
>   McDonald (23), Denhoff and Robinault (43).

A ventriculogram is similar to a pneumoencephalogram except that a ventricular puncture is used to replace the cerebrospinal fluid by air only in the ventricles. The subarachnoid spaces are not made visible by this technique. Both types of intracranial pneumography are hospital procedures.

Skull X Rays

Radiographic examination of the bones of the skull does not require the injection of oxygen into the cavities of the brain. Skull X rays are useful in detecting congenital abnormalities of the skull formation which might interfere with development of the brain. Premature closure of the fontanelles or sutures of the skull with resultant craniostenosis might be detected by a skull X ray. Areas of calcification in the brain may be revealed by roentgenography. This procedure is not useful in diagnosing cerebral palsy but may be employed in identifying other pathological conditions which might be rectified.

These special examinations will not be ordered routinely but only when the clinical examination reveals a need for more detailed studies. More frequently the examining physician is likely to request that the cerebral palsied child be studied by an ophthalmologist and an otologist. These examinations will not be helpful in diagnosing cerebral palsy, but problems of vision and hearing are frequently found in cerebral palsied children.

CLASSIFICATION OF CEREBRAL PALSY

A number of systems for classifying cerebral palsy patients have been developed. Of particular usefulness are those classifications which categorize the cerebral palsied on the basis of neuromuscular characteristics, topography of involvement, and program needs.

Classification on the Basis of Neuromuscular Characteristics

Five major types of cerebral palsy may be identified. These are spasticity, athetosis, tremor, rigidity, and ataxia.

Spasticity

The neuromuscular condition characteristic of spasticity is an increase in the stretch reflex. In addition there is an increase in muscle

25 The normal stretch reflex is essential for maintaining muscle tone and assists in the maintenance of posture. The exaggerated stretch reflexes associated with upper motor neuron lesions cause many of the aberrations of movement and posture seen in cerebral palsy. Compare the neurophysiological bases of the normal and the exaggerated stretch reflexes. See Gardner (61), Fulton (60), Sherrington (164), Granit (69), Chusid and McDonald (23), Magoun (112: 113-27), and (113).

tone of the spastic muscle and a weakness in those muscles which are in opposition to the spastic muscles. Hyperactive stretch reflexes are particularly noticeable in the antigravity muscles, i.e., those muscles which work against gravity in maintaining posture. Clonus may be elicited in any spastic muscle but is most easily demonstrated in the ankle jerk reflex.

Because of the hyperactive stretch reflexes and slow contraction time, the movements of the spastic are poorly coordinated. The tendency for the antigravity muscles to maintain a state of contraction and for the antagonists to lengthen correspondingly produces characteristic flexion deformities, particularly at the large joints. The typical spastic with involvement on one side will show flexion at the wrist and elbow, adduction and internal rotation of the arm, adduction and flexion at the hip, flexion of the knee, and equinus of the foot. There is a small group of spastics called *atonic spastics* whose main neuromuscular characteristic is muscular weakness rather than spasticity. These children do not develop the typical deformities of the spastic and they require different treatment procedures.

Athetosis

The muscle of the athetoid is normal, that is, there is no spasticity nor weakness; however, some athetoids will have traces of spasticity in the lower extremities. The distinguishing characteristic of the athetoid is involuntary movement which occurs with voluntary effort and interferes with normal muscle functions. The involuntary movement may be of one of two types: tremor or rotary, and it may occur with or without tension. Tremor involuntary motions consist of flexion and extension motions of hinge joints. Rotary involuntary motions are the result of involuntary contractions of the muscles around ball-and-socket joints. Tension is a state of contraction of both the agonists and antagonists. It is thought to result from the habituation of efforts to control involuntary motions. Some physicians and therapists feel that this is not a completely adequate explanation of the tension which is seen in some athetoids. In the dystonic athetoid the tension may be so extreme as to incapacitate the patient.

Several clinical types of athetosis have been described, but all of them have the basic involuntary motions of either the tremor or rotary pattern. There is no general agreement about the terminology nor the specific characteristics of the various types of athetoids. In part this

> 26   Athetosis is usually attributed to lesions in the extrapyramidal tract or in the basal ganglia. There is considerable variability in what authors of textbooks in speech pathology, anatomy, and physiology and in neurophysiology include in the basal ganglia. Compare West, Ansberry, and Carr (186), Gardner (61), Kaplan (96), Magoun (112: 113-27), Fulton (60). What are the functions of the basal ganglia?

is because the conditions do not occur frequently enough to give examiners an opportunity to study and classify them. One type of athetoid which is seen less frequently today is the Rh athetoid who, in addition to the involuntary movement patterns, has a high-frequency hearing loss. Under physical and emotional stress the involuntary motions and tension of the athetoid increase. Because the muscle is basically normal and the tension disappears during rest or sleep, characteristic deformities rarely develop in the athetoid.

Ataxia

The ataxic's muscles are normal, although there may at times be some muscular weakness. There is no spasticity nor are there involuntary motions. Reflexes are normal. The distinguishing characteristic of the ataxic is the disturbance of equilibrium. His righting reflex is diminished and his sense of position in space is disturbed. As a rule, ataxia is not diagnosed until the child begins to walk. This is because prior to the disturbed balance which appears when the child begins walking, the only symptom present is hypotonia. Some ataxics improve spontaneously and may even develop normal neuromuscular function; hence, their picture may vary as the child grows older.

> 27   The cerebellum is involved in various phases of synergic muscle action. Cerebellar lesions affect the regularity of muscular action. What are the common disorders of volitional movement associated with cerebellar dysfunction? Fulton (60), Gardner (61), Chusid and McDonald (23), DeJong (39).

Tremor

The muscles of the tremor type of cerebral palsy are normal in tone and there are no abnormal reflexes. The distinguishing neuromuscular characteristic is repetitive, rhythmic involuntary contractions of flexor and extensor muscles. These tremors may be either intentional or nonintentional. Intentional tremors are not present during rest but appear with voluntary or "intended" movement. Nonintentional tremors are present during rest and continue with the intentional movement. The tremor type of cerebral palsy differs from the athetoid type: the involuntary movements of the tremor type are fine and rhythmic, whereas those of the athetoid are gross and variable. Tremors in the lower extremities may throw the patient off balance. Tremors in the upper extremities interfere with the development of hand skills. Some tremors interfere with the performance of precise movements to such a degree that it is impossible for the patient to develop skills such as writing. Often tremors can also be seen in the tongue, especially when protruded. However, the tremor type of cerebral palsy does not develop any deformities.

Rigidity

The distinguishing neuromuscular characteristic of rigidity is a resistance to flexion and extension movements resulting from simultaneous contraction of both the agonist and antagonist muscle groups. Attempts to move a limb are often described as similar to bending a lead pipe. In some cases the rigidity is constant; in other cases it is intermittent. During the intermittent phase the muscles are weak. Reflexes are diminished or absent. All extremities are involved in rigidity because of the generalized disturbance of neuromuscular function. The patient whose rigidity is constant is likely to develop deformities, whereas the intermittent type of rigidity is less likely to result in them. Because of the simultaneous contractions of agonists and antagonists, persons with rigidity are capable only of slow movements within a restricted range.

Mixed

Careful examination of cerebral palsy patients will reveal that some patients exhibit combinations of neuromuscular characteristics. Their over-all appearance will be determined by the type of neuromuscular characteristic which predominates. Spastics, for example, may be found to have some weak, nonspastic, or even normal muscles. In some athetoids mild spasticity can be elicited in the lower extremities. Other combinations are less frequently found, but such patterns as spasticity coexisting with rigidity have been observed.

Classification on the Basis of Topography

Cerebral palsy may also be classified according to the number and location of the limbs which are involved, that is, the topographical distribution of the involvement. The three most commonly used classifications are hemiplegia, paraplegia, and quadriplegia. In paraplegia, both legs are involved, but there is no involvement of the arms. Cerebral palsied persons who are paraplegics are likely to be of the spastic type. Hemiplegics have one arm and one leg involved on the same side of the body. These are most often spastics, but occasionally an athetoid or rigidity hemiplegic is seen. In quadriplegia all four extremities are involved. Quadriplegics may be spastics, athetoids, tremors, rigidities, or ataxics. In diplegia there is involvement of all four extremities; however, the legs are primarily involved and there is only slight involvement of the arms. These cases are usually spastics. In triplegia there is involvement of three extremities, usually two legs and one arm. Some physicians doubt that the one arm is completely normal and are inclined to classify these patients as quadriplegics with one good arm. Monoplegia, that is the involvement of only one limb, is extremely rare. Often cases classified as monoplegics will, after more careful observation, be seen to have either mild paraplegia or mild hemiplegia. Double hemiplegia is used to describe those spastic quadriplegics whose arms are more involved than their legs. Also, as a rule, quadriplegics tend to be about equally involved on both sides; therefore, those who are much more involved on one side than on the other might be classified as double hemiplegics rather than quadriplegics.

Classification on the Basis of the Patient's Needs

Another useful method of classifying individuals who are cerebral palsied is in terms of his program needs. To say that a child is a spastic quadriplegic, for example, gives little information about the kind of program which should be developed for him. Effective planning for any cerebral palsied individual must take into account his

Name: _____

B.D.: _____

Dx: _____

Clinic: _____ Date: _____

	MEDICAL							DENTAL		THERAPIES			PSYCHO-SOCIAL				OTHER CONSIDERATIONS		
	Pediatric	Orthopedic surgery/bracing	Vision	Hearing	Neurologic surgery / special studies	Special Drugs	Psychiatric	General	Special	OT	PT	ST	Testing	Family Counseling	Personal Adjustment Counseling	Vocational Counseling	Environmental Adjustment	Special Equipment	Recreation
EDUCATIONAL PROGRAM																			
HOME PROGRAM — Instruction and treatment (Birth to 3 or 3 1/2 yrs)																			
GROUP PROGRAM — Socialization and instruction (3 1/2 to 6 years)																			
REGULAR CLASS																			
ORTHOPEDIC CLASS a. Mentally normal b. Mentally retarded																			
CLASS FOR RETARDED a. Primary b. Intermediate c. Jr. H. School d. Sr. H. School																			
DAY CARE PROGRAM																			
RESIDENT EDUCATION AND TREATMENT																			
HOME BOUND																			
OTHER SPECIAL EDUCATION																			
VOCATIONAL																			
COMPETITIVE EMPLOYMENT																			
SHELTERED WORKSHOP																			
CARE																			
CUSTODIAL (HOME)																			
CUSTODIAL (RESIDENTIAL)																			

(Side labels: SPREOCHOOL — HOME PROGRAM / GROUP PROGRAM; SCHOOL — REGULAR CLASS through CLASS FOR RETARDED; AGE — DAY CARE PROGRAM through OTHER SPECIAL EDUCATION; SPCOHOOTL — VOCATIONAL; AANGYE — CARE) age, the kind of educational or vocational program most appropriate for him, and the kinds of evaluative and therapeutic services needed to meet his particular problems. How an individual might be classified in terms of his program needs can be seen by inspecting the chart on page 39.

Three important ages shown at the left of the chart are considered. During the early part of the preschool period, the child's program would consist primarily of instruction and treatment carried on at home but supervised closely through regular clinic visits. The later preschool program would consist of group activities stressing socialization and instruction conducted either by a private or public agency. During the school-age period, the child's educational program would be provided in a class appropriate for his physical status and his intellectual ability.

> 28   What are the elements of an adequate educational program for cerebral palsied children at the preschool, elementary-school, and secondary-school levels? What factors determine the type of program each child should have? See Hopkins, Bice, and Cotton (84), Dunsdon (47), Berenberg (9: 27-33), Cruickshank (32). Also see (49).

During the postschool period, the emphasis would shift from an educational program to a vocational program, and the patient might be employed either in a competitive situation or in a sheltered workshop.

For some cerebral palsied patients who are severely impaired in their intellectual functioning, educational and vocational programming will be inappropriate. The program for these children will consist of providing adequate care rather than treatment and education. Initially good care can be provided at home, but for many it eventually becomes advisable to arrange for care in a state institution for the mentally retarded. Educational and vocational programming for the intellectually normal but severely physically involved child will also be difficult and at times inappropriate. At the present time there are few adequate residential centers for such children and most of them must be cared for in their own homes.

The various medical, dental, psychosocial, therapeutic, and other services which a cerebral palsied individual might need are indicated across the top of the chart. In an adequate program for cerebral palsied children, each child's condition would be carefully studied to determine which of these services he would need. His needs and, hence, his classification changes as he grows older or as certain services are completed. The use of such a classification scheme facilitates the coordination of services for a given child and encourages long-term planning of his program. This chart does not indicate the specific kind of treatment a child should have but only the general nature of the treatment. For example, the kind of orthopedic surgery or the kind of bracing would not be important in this classification. However, because surgery or bracing is needed, it would be considered important to categorize this under the child's needs. This would also be true about occupational, physical, and speech therapy. It is not essential when classifying the child to specify the particular techniques to be employed by the therapists. It is enough to know that he needs one or more of these therapies.

Using this approach to classification one can now describe a child in program terms. For example, a child might be classified as a pre-school-age spastic quadriplegic who has been evaluated by the psychologist and who is: (a) participating in a group program of socialization and instruction, (b) wearing braces and receiving special medication, (c) participating in occupational, speech, and physical therapy programs, and (d) using special equipment at home and at school. This information together with the staff's estimate of the overall severity of his involvement provides a meaningful basis for program planning.

When such a chart is carefully completed for all the cerebral palsied individuals in an area, it becomes possible to identify the program needs of the cerebral palsied population at any particular time and to project the needs of this population ahead for several years.

Do we have enough information about Charlene Pimskon to determine the cause of her cerebral palsy? Of what type is it? What is the topography of her involvement? Her birth weight of three pounds indicates that she was premature. Since speech and hand function are normal and only the lower extremities are involved, she is probably a paraplegic. The toe standing, leg scissoring, and ankle clonus are indications of hyperactive stretch reflexes; so, she is probably a spastic paraplegic. In her rehabilitation program, would she need physical therapy? Speech therapy? Occupational therapy? Do her parents need a counseling program? What other services might they need?

What do you think might be the cause of cerebral palsy in each of the other cases? What type of cerebral palsy does each have? Can you determine the topography of involvement for each? What impressions can you form regarding program needs?

IT HAS BEEN ESTIMATED THAT ONE IN EVERY SIXTEEN BABIES BORN IN the United States has a serious defect. Some of these defects are the result of hereditary factors. It has recently been demonstrated that our genes contain a chemical called *DNA* (deoxyribonucleic acid). This substance is actually a chemical code which determines all the inherited characteristics of man.[1] This code is passed along from one generation to another through the genes. Genes are combined in larger structures called *chromosomes*. Some birth defects, e.g., mongolism, have been linked to chromosomal errors. Others, such as phenylketonuria, have been linked to a single mutant gene. Hostile intrauterine chemical environments may also affect the embryologic growth of a child. A number of chemicals which might appear in the unborn child's environment as a result of maternal illness or medication have detrimental

4 *associated problems*

influences on embryonic tissues. Probably a great many birth defects are the result of hereditary and environmental factors operating together. It is thought that hereditary factors may cause a baby to be susceptible to potentially detrimental intrauterine environmental causes, whereas another baby, with a different hereditary background, would not be disturbed by the same environmental conditions. These factors may result in a wide variety of conditions such as skeletal malformations, malformation of organs, mental retardation, visual problems, hearing problems, and many others.

> 29 While some congenital malformations are so gross as to be incompatible with life, others are so mild as to make the borderline between normal and abnormal difficult to establish. What are the common congenital defects which involve the central nervous system? See Fishbein, ed. (*58*) and Chusid and McDonald (*23*).

The cerebral palsied child may, in addition to the factors resulting in his motor disability, have other problems resulting from chromosomal

[1] For a popular discussion of DNA see *Time,* May 23, 1960 and *Life,* November 2, 1962. For a more scientific discussion see Fishbien, ed. (*58*).

errors, mutant genes, hostile intrauterine chemical environment, or combinations of these. Hence, we should be careful not to attribute all of the cerebral palsied child's problems to his cerebral palsy.

Our definition of cerebral palsy has emphasized that the condition is characterized by a motor disability resulting from damage to the brain. We have also emphasized that cerebral palsied individuals are multiply handicapped. Not only might the multiple handicaps be the result of birth defects not directly associated with the condition causing the cerebral palsy, but many of the multiple problems might be the result of damage to the brain which produced the motor disability leading to a diagnosis of cerebral palsy. It is not difficult to see, therefore, why an individual cerebral palsied child might have one or more of the following handicapping conditions.

MENTAL RETARDATION

The term *mental retardation* is preferred to such older terms as feeble-mindedness and mental deficiency. Definitions of mental retardation have been formulated in psychosocial, medical, educational, legal, and other terms. A definition which is particularly helpful to our understanding of this problem in the cerebral palsied is presented in *A Manual on Terminology and Classification in Mental Retardation*.[2] This definition views mental retardation as subaverage general intellectual functioning which originates during the developmental period and is associated with impairment in adaptive behavior. The three aspects of adaptive behavior—maturation, learning, and social adjustment—included in this definition point up the difficulty encountered in assessing the mental status of the cerebral palsied. Maturation is concerned with the development of sitting, crawling, standing, walking, talking, and other self-help skills. Delayed development of these skills is regarded as an important indication of mental retardation. When we consider that these skills require motor coordinations which may be difficult for the cerebral palsied child because of his motor deficit, we realize that delayed development of these skills may not, in his case, be the result of mental retardation, but rather of a motor disability.

In this definition, learning refers to the facility with which knowledge is acquired as a function of experience. Slowness in learning is regarded as an indication of mental retardation. However, because of his motor

---

[2]*American Journal of Mental Deficiency*, Monograph Supplement, September 1961.

disability, the cerebral palsied child has fewer opportunities to interact with his environment and, hence, gains fewer experiences than does the normal child. His reduced opportunities for experiencing may make the cerebral palsied child appear to be mentally retarded. The third aspect of adaptive behavior, social adjustment, has to do with the de-

30   The possibility that experience influences the child's intellectual level has important implications for habilitating the cerebral palsied. What are the bases for the suggestion that skillfully arranged exposures to specialized environments may improve the intellectual functioning of cerebral palsied children? See Hunt (87), Bruner (18: 1-16), Piaget (146), and (178). Compare these views with those of Ilg and Ames (88).

gree of independence which the individual is able to obtain. Again, there are many factors other than intellectual potential which interfere with the development of independence by cerebral palsied individuals.

These comments are intended to point up the difficulties in assessing the intellectual potential of cerebral palsied children. They should not be construed to mean that their potential cannot be assessed or that most cerebral palsied children are mentally normal but appear to be retarded because of their motor handicap. As a matter of fact, several

31   Standardized testing procedures are sometimes inappropriate for assessing the intellectual potential of cerebral palsied children. What procedures are employed by psychologists in testing cerebral palsied children at different age levels? See Taylor (176), Hausserman (79: 2-23), Miller and Rosenfield (117: 613-21), and Allen and Jefferson (2).

carefully conducted investigations concur that most cerebral palsied children suffer some degree of intellectual impairment. Only about 25 per cent may be classified as normal or above normal. Approximately 30 per cent are slightly retarded and the remaining 45 per cent must be classified as moderately or severely retarded. Those in the borderline group might be regarded as educable mentally retarded children, whereas those in the moderate or severe group would be regarded as trainable mentally retarded children.

These figures should not be surprising. More than ninety factors have been identified as potential causes of mental retardation. Any of these might operate to impair the intellectual function of the child who also has cerebral palsy. Then, too, we must remember that his brain damage is seldom so selective that only one function is impaired. As a rule the brain damage affects intellectual potential as well as motor abilities of cerebral palsied children. For many years it was felt that athetoids had intellectual ability superior to that of spastics because the athetoids' lesions were subcortical and the spastics' lesions were in the cerebral cortex. Recent comparisons of spastics and athetoids suggest that the differences between the two groups are probably not significant. In our experience the topography of the involvement is more likely to be related to intellectual status than the type of cerebral palsy. The spastics do not constitute a homogeneous group, and the spastic paraplegics are least likely to have intellectual deficits. Mental retardation is somewhat more likely to be found among the hemiplegics; an even greater proportion of spastic quadriplegics are likely to suffer some degree of mental retardation.

It is difficult to generalize about mental retardation in cerebral palsy. First there is the problem of separating the effects of severe motor disability from the effects of retarded intellectual development. Second, it must be remembered that there are many subgroups among the cerebral palsied, and that these subgroups may not be represented in the same proportion in every treatment center. In our experience an important approach to assessing the intellectual potential of a cerebral palsied child is to evaluate his progress in therapeutic and educational situations.

For severely handicapped children, psychological testing establishes a baseline which gives the therapist and teacher some notion of where to start treating and teaching the child. To the information provided by the psychological test, knowledgeable and observant therapists and teachers can add information which will aid the treatment group in determining to what extent a child's slow progress may be attributed to his motor disability and to what degree his progress is influenced by his intellectual development. Not only will this approach result in an assessment which is more fair to the child, but it will also make any forthcoming diagnosis of mental retardation more acceptable to his parents.

HEARING

Again it is to be noted that factors which might produce a hearing loss in any child may be potential causes of auditory impairment in the cerebral palsied. Clinical experience strongly suggests however that the incidence of auditory impairment is much higher among cerebral palsied children than it is in the general population of children.

32   Review the findings of the New Jersey study (84) and the reports of Rutherford (156: 237-40) and Fisch (57: 370-71) on the incidence of hearing loss in cerebral palsied children. What are the implications of the articles by Hardy (77: 3-7), Asher (5: 475-77), and Byers, Paine, and Crothers (19: 248-53) for the interpretation of incidence studies?

Once again we have difficulty interpreting the results of surveys reporting the hearing status of children classified by a type of cerebral palsy. Often they make no distinctions among subgroups on the basis of topography or severity of involvement. Estimates of hearing losses have ranged from as low as 10 per cent to over 30 per cent of the cerebral palsied population. Some of these differences may be attributed to differing definitions of hearing loss and differing methods of testing. Probably an even greater source of the difference lies in the differences among the populations studied.

More important than the numbers of children with hearing losses is information about the types of loss a therapist might encounter. Many athetoids with a history of Rh incompatibility are found to have a high-frequency hearing loss which is overlooked during their early life, because they respond to noises and to many sounds. Not until it is noted that they have difficulty differentiating between sounds and particularly that they are having difficulty in developing speech is a hearing loss suspected. Central deafness may also be found among athetoids with a history of kernicterus. In these children the peripheral auditory structures found in the outer, middle, and inner ear are intact, but lesions have occurred in various parts of the central auditory mechanism due to the kernicterus. Central hearing losses might occur in other cerebral palsied children as a result of damage to cortical hearing centers. Many therapists insist that some cerebral palsied children show intermittent hearing losses or variable auditory acuity which cannot be attributed to infections of the upper respiratory tract or to a temporary middle-ear pathology. The existence of such intermittent hearing losses has not been established, but as a phenomenon it deserves continued observation and study.

The therapist can be especially helpful in determining the auditory status of cerebral palsied children. While it is usually easy to assess the hearing of mildly cerebral palsied children employing standardized hearing techniques, these techniques are less applicable to the severely involved child. The electroencephalogram and the psychogalvanic skin-response test have been used with children who cannot be tested by standard approaches. These techniques are not available to a great many clinics. The validity of psychogalvanic responses as a measure of auditory functioning in the cerebral palsied has been questioned because it is felt that the damaged nervous system of the cerebral palsied child would not be capable of the neurophysiological functioning required in psychogalvanic testing. Important information about the child's auditory functioning may evolve from the careful and skilled observations of therapists and teachers. Until there is evidence to prove otherwise, *therapists and teachers should suspect every cerebral palsied child of having a hearing loss.* All the professional workers associated with cerebral palsied children should be familiar with the behavioral signs of hearing impairment and should constantly be on the lookout for these signs when working with cerebral palsied children.

EMOTIONAL PROBLEMS

An early point of view about the personality development of the cerebral palsied held that personalities of the five major types of cerebral palsy differed so greatly that a diagnosis of the physical condition could be made by observing the personality. According to this point of view, spastics were viewed as the direct opposites of athetoids. Whereas spastics were introverts, fearful, and slow to anger, athetoids were regarded as extroverts, fearless, and quick to anger. The emotional characteristics of the ataxic were described as similar to those of athetoids but with distinguishable differences.

Careful observations of cerebral palsied children did not support this point of view and it now seems more likely that the behavior

33   Compare the points of view of Phelps (*141*: 3-5) and Garmezy
     (*62*: 348-55).

patterns and attitudes of cerebral palsied children are determined to a large extent by the nature of their experiences during their early years. Because the cerebral palsied child has difficulty in getting about, in caring for himself, in talking to others, and in doing for others, he does not experience normal opportunities for emotional growth. His delayed maturation may result in a failure to develop drives which constitute motivating forces for normal children. His feelings of personal worth

34   It has been suggested that if socialization opportunities are delayed
     beyond the fifth year of life for the cerebral palsied child, severe emo-
     tional damage will result. What is the normal pattern of social de-
     velopment during this period and why does the cerebral palsied child
     have difficulty following these maturational sequences? See Gesell (*63*)
     and Bice (*12*: 120-31).

are never reinforced and he may eventually draw the conclusion that he is an inferior person. Since he has little opportunity to develop his interests, he learns to live with a minimum of interests. When the cerebral palsied child learns that, with minimum effort on his part, his basic needs will be met, he often becomes satisfied with minimum effort and his functioning levels off at the point which serves his immediate needs. When the responsibility for decision making rests not with him but with the adults in his environment, he fails to develop beyond an infantile level.

Unfavorable parental attitudes also adversely affect the emotional development of the cerebral palsied child. There are parents who deny that any disability exists and live in hope that "everything will be all right." Their children are not likely to be objective about their limitations. Well intentioned parents are often overprotective about their cerebral palsied child. They do not want him to be hurt physically or emotionally and they do not require of him anything which would call for considerable effort on his part. Immaturity and dependency are engendered by this type of parental attitude. Rejection is a common and natural reaction of parents to a severely handicapped child. The child's response is to become withdrawn and insecure.

These attitudes have a harmful effect on the cerebral palsied child's development. In some children the psychological and emotional problems are so severe that the child is unable to benefit from the treatment and educational programs. Many cerebral palsied adults are lacking in the drive to do even the things they are capable of doing. They seem to have no goals in life, or, often, the goals they have are unrealistic. The adult life of many cerebral palsied persons is dominated by fear—fear of failure, of meeting people, of injury and accident, of being alone. Often these fears are out of line with reality. The emotional problems of many cerebral palsied adults constitute greater obstacles to employment than does their physical disability.

> 35 It is quite easy for a therapist to become so concerned about the cerebral palsied child's difficulties that the problems of the child's parents are overlooked. What feelings naturally arise when a handicapped child is part of a family and what happens if these feelings are not understood and managed? See McDonald (108), Bice (11), Denhoff and Holden (41: 5-7), Wortis (192: 8-9).

Friends, neighbors, casual acquaintances react in a variety of ways to the cerebral palsied individual. Some are curious; others pity him. Many are overly solicitous; some are even fearful of him. All these reactions have an influence on the developing self-concept of the child with cerebral palsy.

We have seen some adolescent cerebral palsied persons whose severe emotional disturbances were traceable not only to the long-term efforts of parents, but also to the efforts of therapists whose job it was to motivate the child during the many years he was under treatment. Indirectly—and often very directly—we suggest to the child that, as a result of treatment, he will learn to walk, or talk, or feed himself, or whatever we happen to be trying to teach him. Everyone, in talking with the cerebral palsied child, places great value on such skills as walking, talking, and self-help. When the severely involved child (usually in adolescence when he encounters many other problems of adjustment) becomes aware that for him these are unattainable goals, the seed of emotional turmoil, which we inadvertently sowed and nourished, quickly develops into a malformed plant.

Therapists can do much to assist the cerebral palsied child achieve a more wholesome mental hygiene. First they must recognize that some of the responsibility for guiding the child's emotional development rests with them. Meeting the emotional needs of cerebral palsied children is not solely the obligation of parents and counselors. Therapists should educate parents to the dangers of overprotectiveness as well as find ways to give the child some responsibility for making decisions. Parents and therapists together should help the child recognize and capitalize on any capabilities that he possesses so that he can begin to develop a feeling of personal worth. Motivational efforts should be concentrated on short-term goals rather than on long-range goals which may prove unattainable for the cerebral palsied child. Above all, parents and therapists must be aware from the beginning that personality adjustment is not achieved through a "talking to" or a series of discussions in adolescence. Optimal emotional adjustment is best attained through careful attention to the child's emotional needs throughout his life.

DISTURBANCES OF TACTILE AND KINESTHETIC FUNCTIONS

Since the early 1950's there has been a growing interest in: (a) the effects of sensory stimulation on motor function, (b) the effects of sensory deprivation on intellectual and perceptual development, and (c) the nature of sensory disturbances in cerebral palsied children. In fact, a current quip has it that everyone is now talking "sense." Earlier, researchers and therapists were preoccupied with the nature of the motor output, but now they recognize that to a large degree what comes out depends on what goes in.

In Chapter II we described sensory-motor activity as the function of a reaction mechanism consisting of receptors, nervous system, and effectors. Receptors function to activate and to monitor the output of the effectors. Tactile and proprioceptive stimuli are essential to the initiation of postural reflexes and righting reactions and to the control of movement.

There is increasing evidence that many children with cerebral palsy have disturbances of tactile sensitivity and tactile perception. Hemiplegics, who have no difficulty identifying objects placed in their normal hand, cannot identify the same objects when they are placed in the neurologically disturbed hand. There are hints that walkers and nonwalkers among the cerebral palsied may differ in the level of the pain threshold in the foot. It has often been pointed out that an extensor reflex of the lower extremity is commonly elicited in cerebral palsied children who do not walk and that a similar extensor pattern is found in the early walking attempts of the normal child. The presence of this extensor reflex may be related to the hypersensitivity of the forefoot. There are indications, too, that some cerebral palsied children differ from normal children in their ability to identify forms placed in their mouths and that their defective oral sensory functions are related to defective motor performances in chewing, drinking, and articulating.

36   What are the implications of the work of Tizard (*179*: 628-32), Hohman Baker, and Reed (*83*: 1-6), Wiedenbaker (*190*: 603-10), and Solomon (*168*) for the treatment of cerebral palsied children? What further studies should be done in this area?

We know of no studies of proprioceptive function in the cerebral palsied, but it appears obvious that the stimuli received from muscles in a state of exaggerated stretch reflexes or from muscles producing tremors would be very different from the sensations associated with normal movements. It would seem logical to expect that such bizarre sensory inputs would have a detrimental influence on motor learning.

Deprivation of visual and auditory stimuli can produce significant disturbances of intellectual and perceptual processes in normals. Reduction of tactile-kinesthetic stimulation without interfering with visual and auditory functions impairs intellectual functioning in normal male subjects. While there are obvious dangers in applying these findings to cerebral palsied children, we cannot overlook the hint that perhaps some of their apparent intellectual and perceptual impairments may be due to sensory deprivation or sensory malfunction. Further, the importance assigned to exteroceptive stimulation in arousing and maintaining man's motivation suggests a possible relationship between the defective sensory function and the low motivational level of some cerebral palsied children. Most of these comments are speculative, for very little is known about the nature of sensory functioning in the cerebral palsied or the effects of sensory malfunctioning. Strong evidence seems to be developing that defective sensory functioning may in part be responsible for the defective motor functioning characteristic of the cerebral palsied. There are also hints that defective sensory functioning may have a detrimental influence on intelligence, perception, and personality development.

> 37   Are some cerebral palsied children being brainwashed from birth? Studies of the effects of sensory deprivation, which is one of the techniques of brainwashing, suggest that some of the problems of brain-damaged children might be due to sensory deprivation. What are these effects and how may they be counteracted? See Zubek and Wilgosh (*194:* 306-308). Solomon *et. al.* (*169*), Hebb (*80:* 109-14), Bexton, Heron, and Scott (*10:* 70-76).

ORTHOPEDIC PROBLEMS IN CEREBRAL PALSY

The cerebral palsied child may have any orthopedic problem which any other child might have—clubfoot, congenital deformities of the spine, and so forth. These problems are not necessarily the result of his being cerebral palsied. There are, however, several orthopedic problems seen in cerebral palsied populations which *are* the result of muscle malfunction. Flexor deformities due to spasticity occur in both the upper and lower extremities. Knee-flexion deformities as seen in the bent-knee gait are common. Flexor deformities are also seen at the hip, elbow, and wrist. Another example of this type of deformity is seen in the thumb-in-palm and flexed-finger posture associated with the spastic.

Abnormal postural attitudes and deformities may result from muscular weakness. Badly pronated feet may be due to inactive tibial muscles. Weak spinal muscles may lead to loss of normal lordosis. Head drop may result from weak posterior neck muscles. The flexed position associated with loss of normal lordosis and weak abdominal muscles may lead to flaring of the rib margins.

Abnormal muscle stresses may produce changes in the architecture of certain bones. For a short time the normal child sits with his feet behind him, but he soon learns to stand and walk. The cerebral palsied child is apt to maintain this sitting position for years because it gives him a broader base for sitting support. In this position there is an internal femoral torsion which may produce as much as 45 degrees of twisting in the femoral bone. This twisting will result in a toeing-in gait when the child begins to walk. The tibia may become externally rotated on the femur and the knee ligaments markedly relaxed because of an abnormal sitting position. Children with this condition tend to stand with their knees together and the knee caps internally rotated.

One of the most common orthopedic problems encountered in cerebral palsy is dislocation of one or both hips. The normal infant tends to lie in the "frog position," that is, with the thighs abducted and externally rotated in relation to the pelvis and hip sockets. This position helps to produce normal architectural relationships between the head of the femur and the hip socket. Development of a deep hip socket is encouraged by this relationship. In the normal child balanced strength in the abductors and adductors tend to pull the femur into the hip socket. In the cerebral palsied child there is often a weakness in the abductors and spasticity in the adductors and hamstrings. This creates a situation which is the opposite of the frog position. There is a tendency for these abnormal muscle pulls to push the head of the thigh bone out and up from the socket. The congenitally dislocated hip seen in non-cerebral-palsied children is usually the result of an osseous deformity. The dislocated hip seen in the cerebral palsied child is usually the result of neuromuscular malfunction. Because of the frequency of this condition, it is important to have yearly X rays of the hips of children who tend to scissor.

Therapists, particularly speech and occupational therapists, are often desirous of having the child sit in a stable position during speech therapy or feeding training. Unless care is exercised to prevent the child from sitting with his feet behind him, the stabilization sought for speech and occupational therapy might lead to the development of an orthopedic deformity.

While a dislocated hip is a serious but correctable handicap for the non-cerebral-palsied child, for the child whose neuromuscular malfunction is severe enough to produce a dislocated hip the dislocated hip is but a minor additional handicap. It should be noted, too, that a hip dislocated by abnormal muscle forces will not respond to the same corrective treatment as does the congenitally dislocated hip. It is important, however, that the condition be recognized and, if possible, anticipated so that the parents will not worry unduly about it. In most instances a dislocated hip in a cerebral palsied child does not call for treatment, and its presence should not interfere with positioning the child during some of the treatment procedures.

VISUAL PROBLEMS IN CEREBRAL PALSY

It is to be remembered that the cerebral palsied child might have any of the ocular problems which non-cerebral-palsied children might have. In addition there are some visual defects which occur commonly in cerebral palsy. Some problems result from imbalances of the extra-ocular muscles. Normally these muscles position the eyes so that the image transmitted from each eye to the occipital lobe is blended into one image rather than represented as two separate images. This blending results in stereoscopic vision. If the two images do not blend, *diplopia,* or double vision, occurs. The brain will not tolerate diplopia and suppresses one of the images. The eye providing that image eventually becomes blind, a condition called *amblyopia.* This loss of vision is not due to any visible pathology in the eye itself but rather to a condition in the brain. In the young, normal child it is natural for one or the other of the eyes to deviate in the horizontal plane. This condition, known as an *alternating squint,* disappears as the child matures. In the cerebral palsied child, however, the condition remains as a *fixed squint.* When the eye deviates toward the nose, the condition is known as *esotropia.* When the eye deviates away from the nose, the condition is known as *exotropia.* This condition is also referred to as *strabismus* or *squint.* Treatment may consist of alternate "patching" of the eyes or surgery may be employed to bring the muscular forces into better balance. Lenses may also be used in certain cases. It is important that this condition be treated early because if the child suppresses vision in one eye for several years, blindness will ensue in that eye.

Nystagmus, a to-and-fro movement of the eyes, is also seen in cerebral palsied children. If this condition is present at birth, it is likely that subnormal vision will result. When the nystagmus is of small amplitude, normal vision may develop.

Loss of vertical eye motions is seen in children with histories of kernicterus as in the Rh athetoid. This condition does not impair vision but affects the range of sight. In order to see up or down, the child must tilt the head in the appropriate direction. Fortunately this type of cerebral palsy is now preventable and is seen much less frequently than it was even a few years ago.

Hemianopsia, a loss of half of the visual field of each eye, is seen in some cerebral palsied individuals. Children with hemianopsia will not see objects placed in the area of their defective field of vision. Hemianopsia is found in children who have had hemispherectomies.

Another problem which was seen commonly in premature infants a few years ago was blindness resulting from retrolental fibroplasia. Since the relationship between high oxygen content in the incubator and this disease has been established, it has been possible to prevent this type of blindness in premature children.

Therapists should be careful about the placement of materials for

38   It is difficult to assess the vision of young cerebral palsied children. How
      does the ophthalomologist examine cerebral palsied children and what
      problems does he find most frequently? See Guibor (13: 333-39), (74:
      852-56) and Schacht et al. (157: 623-28).

children with known visual-field defects. If a child consistently fails
to respond to materials the therapist is using, she should consider the
possibility that some type of visual defect is the cause of his failure to
respond to the materials. Children with nystagmus have difficulty
focusing on materials and may need a longer exposure time than
children with normal vision would require. Further, the therapist
should be aware that a child may assume abnormal sitting postures
in order to bring his eyes into comfortable focus on materials which
he wants to see.

SEIZURES

The brain in a way may be viewed as a highly specialized biochemi-
cal plant which converts chemicals found in the body to electrical
voltages. Normally these voltages are liberated in finely graded
quantities and are channeled in a precisely regulated manner over
neuronal pathways. Mechanical, thermal, electrical, or chemical forces
may interfere with the manner in which the brain cells release their
energy. When the brain cells produce excessive voltages, or the rhythm
with which the voltages are channeled over the neuronal pathways is
disturbed, seizures may result. It is not unusual for normal children,
particularly in early life, to have one or two convulsive attacks. These
are usually in conjunction with severe illness and high fever. These
single episodes rarely require continued anticonvulsant therapy.
Cerebral palsied children may have seizures under these conditions.
Because many cerebral palsied children have suffered damage to their
brains, they are likely to have recurrent convulsions. Histories of
seizures are common in spastics, but athetoids are not so likely to have
convulsive episodes. Some spastics without a history of seizures have
abnormal electroencephalograms and may have subclinical seizures.

39   What is the relationship of EEG findings and histories of convulsions to
      type and topography of cerebral palsy? See Perlstein, Gibbs, and Gibbs
      (140: 377-84), Aird and Cohen (1: 448-54).

Types of Seizures

There are several types of convulsions. The *grand mal* type is
characterized by a loss of consciousness, and if the patient is standing

or sitting, he will fall. There may be a period of tonic muscular contractions which is followed by a clonic convulsion. These rapid contractions of the muscles produce vigorous movements of the extremities. Sometimes there is foaming at the mouth. These attacks are usually followed by confusion and lethargy with the child falling asleep for varying lengths of time. For a child subject to grand mal seizures, anticonvulsant therapy must take precedence over all other aspects of the treatment program because it is difficult to treat a child who has frequent periods of unconsciousness and lethargy.

Some convulsive attacks are momentary in nature and may be manifested as single jerks of the head or body or limbs. In these *petit mal* attacks, the child briefly loses contact with his environment. Often these attacks come with great frequency and interfere with the child's progress because his alertness is constantly being interrupted.

In another type of seizure, there is no loss of consciousness nor no generalized convulsive movement. Rather, the jerking is confined to a specific limb. When the convulsive movement starts in one part of the limb and progressively includes more of the body, it is known as a *Jacksonian* seizure.

Subclinical seizures also occur in which there is no outward manifestation of the convulsion. Nevertheless, the brain cells are firing in a paroxysmal rather than in a regulated manner. These seizures were undetected until electroencephalographic studies revealed abnormal brainwave tracings. Therapists should suspect subclinical seizures in children who demonstrate variable attention span and variable performance. Through the use of anticonvulsant medications, it is possible to control a large percentage of cerebral palsied children's seizures.

40   Until recent years epileptic seizures were viewed as the work of devils and epileptics were hidden away. How has this view changed? For a popular discussion see (50) and for a scientific discussion see Penfield and Japser (135).

Not all children respond in the same way to medications. Often children with similar seizure patterns will not respond to the same drug or combination of drugs. It is sometimes necessary, therefore, to try many different drugs in various combinations and dosages in order to discover an effective anticonvulsant regime. Sometimes the drug program required for seizure control may produce excessive drowsiness in the child. Obviously such a program of medication would interfere with the child's therapy program because it is difficult to teach a somnambulant child. For those children whose severe seizures do not respond to anticonvulsant medication, neurosurgery including subtotal hemispherectomies may be advised.

The therapist should be alert for the occurrence of seizures and report them promptly to the appropriate staff member.

DISTURBANCES OF BODY IMAGE

Occasionally cerebral palsied children will be seen who, when told to bend their knees in order to sit in a wheelchair, seem not to know where their knees are located. It has been necessary to heighten their awareness of their body parts before they could be taught to move them appropriately for sitting. Similarly children are seen who seem to be unaware of whether their lips are approximated or their mouths open. Some children are unable to say whether their arms or legs are extended or flexed. They may have difficulty imitating movements or in moving various parts of the body upon command. In adults who have suffered brain damage, this condition is referred to as *body agnosia,* or a loss of the body schema.

Some cerebral palsied children have difficulty developing an adequate

41   How does one develop a body image and what is the relationship of
      body image to personality development and motor function? See Schilder
      (*158*), Fisher (*59*), Bender and Silver (*8:* 84-89).

body image from birth. This is due in part to their disordered tactile and proprioceptive sensory functions. Another source of the child's difficulty in building up a body image is his limited capability for moving his body and for changing the position of his body. Since a severely involved cerebral palsied child has few opportunities for sitting down and getting up by himself, he does not learn how much he has to bend his knees and his hips in order to assume the proper position to make adequate contact with a chair. If he has been fed all his life by another person, he has had little opportunity to learn where his hand is in relation to food or in relation to his mouth. We suspect that some cerebral palsied children have found the sensory stimuli arising from their aberrant motions and abnormal postures so confusing that they have learned to ignore the sensations. Perhaps as much as the brain suppresses the vision from one eye in diplopia, the brain also ignores confusing sensory input from other modalities. Failure to develop an adequate body image can constitute a serious obstacle to learning movement patterns. Therapeutic efforts directed toward developing self-help skills may be futile if the child is not first made aware of

the existence of the various parts of his body, the location of the
various body parts, and the sensations associated with movements and
positions of the parts.

Development of a body image is also related to the emergence of a
self-concept. The infant's awareness of himself as an individual distinct
from his environment probably begins with an awareness that the hand
is part of him but that the bottle or rattle held in the hand is not. Self-
identification grows as he makes more and more differentiation between
himself and his environment. Experience with handicapped adults
suggests that alterations in their body image resulting from amputa-
tion of, or injury to, a body part often brings undesirable modifications
in their self-concept. It would seem important for therapists and other
professional workers to give greater consideration to the possible relationship between the cerebral palsied child's difficulty in developing
an adequate body image and his later personal adjustment.

DISTURBANCES OF PERCEPTION

As indicated in our discussion of the reaction mechanism, the receptors respond to appropriate stimuli by transmitting sensory impulses to the brain. These impulses give rise to sensation. The organism
is aware of the presence of a stimulus and, since each receptor responds
only to a specific type of stimulus, the organism can identify the type
of stimulus present. A higher-level process, discrimination, enables the
organism to respond to differences between stimuli-arousing sensations
in the same sensory modality. A still higher mental process, perception,
is the means by which the organism gives meaning and significance to
sensations. Perceptions are associated with each modality. We develop
visual perceptions, auditory perceptions, and tactile-motor perceptions.
Rarely, however, does a child receive an isolated stimulus which im-
pinges on only one sensory modality. Toys are seen, felt, and often
heard simultaneously. Foods are seen, felt, tasted, and smelled. Even
the stimuli affecting one modality occur simultaneously with many
other competing stimuli of the same type. A word on a printed page
is surrounded by many other words on that page and the book itself is
part of a large number of visual stimuli. The speech which a child
hears is only a portion of the auditory stimuli simultaneously impinging
on his ear. The tactile-motor sensations associated with writing or
drawing, for example, are only a small portion of the total pattern
of sensations associated with these acts. There are also sensations
associated with maintaining the body posture, and with the changing

of head position as the writing or drawing progresses. Most children learn to focus their attention on the central stimulus and to give only secondary attention to other stimuli present. The ability to keep figure and background stimuli in proper relationship is essential to learning.

Many brain-damaged children find it difficult to respond selectively

42   How may perceptual difficulties be identified in cerebral palsied children and what are their educational implications? See Cruickshank, Bice, and Wallen (31), Zuk (195: 256-59), Robinault (150: 1-6), Strauss and Kephart (172), Strauss and Lehtinen (173).

to a mass of stimuli. Oftentimes they are not able to separate the figure from the background. Adults frequently and easily shift the figure-ground relationship as they give their attention first to one stimulus and then to another. While listening to a conversation in a living room, we become aware of footsteps approaching. We listen as they pass the house, giving only half an ear to the conversation. When it is clear that the walker is not stopping, we easily shift our full attention back to the conversation. We can be concentrating on a page we are reading, quickly shift our visual focus to an apple we are eating and, after taking a bite of the apple, immediately become immersed again in the visual stimuli from the book. While doing this we may be oblivious to the TV in the next room, the conversation in the hall, the room temperature, and the sensations arising from having our left leg thrown across our right knee.

Some cerebral palsied children are unable to shift their attention effectively from one stimulus to another. They become confused by the large number of stimuli present and often seem to be responding to many stimuli simultaneously. When shown line drawings of common objects embedded in drawn backgrounds, the normal child has no difficulty in identifying the object. On the other hand many brain-damaged children have difficulty identifying the drawing, apparently because they are forced to respond to the entire pattern of stimuli present and hence can't respond selectively to the figure. Visual motor tasks such as drawing a diamond or reproducing designs with colored blocks or marbles are difficult for many brain-damaged children.

Perceptual disturbances are not generalized in the cerebral palsied population. Many cerebral palsied children have no difficulty with perceptual function. If a cerebral palsied child has difficulty with perception, he usually does not experience the difficulty in all modalities. A child might have difficulty with figure-background relationships in the visual area but will have no demonstrable difficulty in auditory function.

The importance of knowledge concerning a child's perceptual functioning for the planning of therapy is obvious. If a child is compulsively responsive to many of the visual stimuli present in a situation, steps must be taken to reduce the stimuli present or to desensitize him to all but the central stimulus. If a child cannot respond effectively to a central auditory stimulus because he is distracted by all the other sound present, he must be helped to develop selective listening before he can make effective use of his auditory modality in learning.

Now let us think again about the cerebral palsied people with whom we became acquainted in Chapter I. What indications of associated problems do you find in their histories? Carl Pednok obviously has an orthopedic problem involving his right arm and right leg. His inability to identify objects placed in his right hand makes one suspect astereognosis. What do you make of his periodic losses of consciousness? Are there any other suggestions in Carl's history of associated problems which should be studied further? What do you find in the histories of Charles, Clayton, Catherine, and Charleen which might be suggestive of mental retardation, emotional disturbances, visual difficulties, hearing impairments, perceptual dysfunction, tactile-kinesthetic disturbances, seizures, and orthopedic problems?   ꙮꙮꙮ

Because the cerebral palsied individual always is multiply handicapped, successful treatment of his problems demands the attention of persons possessing many different kinds of training and experience. It is virtually impossible for any one professional worker to assess adequately all the problems or to carry out all the necessary treatment. While physicians employ specific treatments for some of the problems of the cerebral palsied individual, such as seizure control or surgical correction of deformities, physicians do not actually treat cerebral palsied children. Nor does the psychologist treat cerebral palsied children, though he might use some special forms of psychotherapy for certain cerebral palsied individuals. The actual "laying on of hands" is done by therapists. It is the physical, occupational, and speech therapists and the teachers who have the essential and

5 *therapists and therapies*

crucial contacts with the cerebral palsied individual and his parents. Treatment, however, comprises only one portion of the therapist's responsibility.

Observing and Reporting

Physicians, psychologists, and other specialists working alone cannot adequately determine the cerebral palsied individual's deficits. They find it difficult to assess his potential without information gained from day-by-day observations of the child's development and his response to certain treatment procedures. Herein lies one of the most important roles of the therapist in providing an adequate program for the cerebral palsied.

The therapist must know how to observe children, must recognize the significance of what is observed. He must also know how to communicate the pertinent information to physicians, psychologists, and other professional workers who, by training and experience, are qualified to integrate this information.

There are several obstacles to successful fulfillment of this second role. The first obstacle is related to status. To be successful in carrying out the role of observer and reporter, the therapist must recognize that tradition gives to the other professions certain status roles. He must accept the fact that status hierarchies exist. While many professional persons have no difficulty accepting information and suggestions from persons with "less professional status" than they possess, one always encounters certain professional people who feel too threatened to accept the information and aid available. When such a situation exists, a therapist or teacher can completely vitiate the information reported by not being aware of the professional status problems involved. For example, if a therapist reports at a staff meeting certain observations which strongly suggest that an earlier professional opinion was wrong, the natural defensiveness of the consultant might be aroused. Talking it over with him first and, perhaps, letting him have the first opportunity to present the information to the group often solves the problem. It is the child who is important.

A second obstacle to effective reporting is the natural tendency of therapists to become emotionally involved with the problems of their children. The multiplicity of their handicaps and their resulting dependency make cerebral palsied children the recipients of sympathy, maternal feelings, or other subjective reactions from their therapist and teachers. Reports colored by the therapist's emotional involvement with the child are worthless to consultants who need to evaluate and devise an effective program for the child. They also reduce the level of professional status which the consultant is willing to grant to the therapist.

Still another obstacle to adequate reporting and observing is the natural reluctance to be pessimistic about a child's achievement or potential. Everyone associated with a cerebral palsied child is hopeful that he will prove to be educable and treatable. Sometimes this hopefulness becomes wishful thinking and, in the eyes of the therapist, the child seems to be learning and achieving more than can be confirmed by a realistic appraisal.

Beginning therapists sometimes have difficulty working with a professional group because they think that the only legitimate reason for scheduling any treatment for a cerebral palsied child is because the child will be helped by the treatment. The role of these therapists in the group may be weakened because they feel it is unethical for a rehabilitation group to treat a child if the treatment does not promise some improvement in his status. Actually a professional group might decide to treat a child with a poor prognosis for many valid reasons including the following: (*a*) because they are undecided about the child's status and need more information, (*b*) the child offers an opportunity for the professional group to learn more about cerebral palsy, (*c*) scheduling the child provides the only open avenue for counseling the parents, and (*d*) scheduling a particular child might enable the group to establish desirable relationships with a professional worker or agency in the community.

> 43   Reports of observations and findings concerning cerebral palsied children, whether presented orally to a group or as a written statement, should be precise, reliable, and as comprehensive as possible. How can the therapist achieve these objectives in reporting? See Johnson, Darley, and Spriestersbach (92) and Snidecor (167: 67-70).

Therapists must learn that their role includes a responsibility to provide other professional workers with significant and accurate information about the child. To detect items of potential significance, therapists must be able to make observations which seemingly are outside their field of special interests. For example, information about the separation of a child's parents is significant to consultants whether it is provided by a social worker or by a therapist. Evidence of a poorly developed body image or of distorted perceptual function might more easily be obtained by the therapist than by the psychologist. An observant therapist might detect involuntary motion which had not been observed during the initial examination. In working with a cerebral palsied child each worker must realize that he sees the child's problem from a different vantage point. His point of view is determined by his professional training and experience. Also, the conditions under which the child is observed may also determine what is seen and by whom. Therapists and teachers see cerebral palsied children more frequently than do physicians and psychologists. They can also make important observations which physicians and psychologists are not trained or do not have time to make. On the other hand, the physician and psychologist are likely to see more cerebral palsied patients than the therapists, and, hence, they can bring greater breadth and depth of training and experience to the problem. Everyone remembers the difficulties encountered by the traditional group of visually handicapped adult males attempting to employ taxonomic principles in their encounter with a pachyderm. It was not until someone integrated the bits of information supplied by each member of the group that the animal's identity

44 In our version the men are cerebral palsied and their visual defects are associated with this condition. One has retrolental fibroplasia, a second has a congenital slow nystagmus of wide amplitude with resultant myopia and the third has suffered a loss of one-half of the visual field. Describe these conditions and tell with what type of cerebral palsy they are likely to be associated. See Guibor (74: 852-56), Schacht (157: 623-28), Tizard (179: 628-32).

was established. When professional workers pool the observations they have made about a cerebral palsied child, the final evaluation is more than a summing up of these observations. The final evaluation must represent an integration of all available data. Interpretation and integration usually require training and experience beyond that which most beginning therapists possess. The role of the therapist, then, is not to name the animal, nor is it his responsibility to integrate all the available information; his obligation is to provide—and help interpret—data which will lead to adequate program planning.

A therapist who envisions her role as consisting solely of treating children will regard the child's progress as an important indicator of her excellence as a therapist. With this orientation there is a strong tendency to see progress where it has not occurred or to overestimate the amount of progress which has been attained. The therapist who envisions the objective reporting of significant observations as an important aspect of her role will avoid this trap. She will not feel compelled to report progress where there is no progress in order to satisfy her personal needs or the needs of administrators or other professional staff members. When a group is developing or trying out a new method, objectivity in evaluating progress is especially essential, yet, it is just at such a time that one's scientific attitude is most easily set aside. Clinical competence involves not only the ability to help a child develop new skills, but also the ability to assess objectively his progress and potential and to report this accurately even when the report is pessimistic. Probably no other problem in rehabilitation places a greater obligation for accurate observing and reporting on the therapist than does the program for the cerebral palsied.

APPROACHES TO THERAPY

Quite naturally the reader now expects to be told *how* to treat cerebral palsied children. Unfortunately, on this subject there is neither unanimity of opinion nor uniformity of methodology. Many methods for treating cerebral palsied children have been proposed. The strongest supporters of each method are the originators of the method, their students, and those parents whose children seem to have been aided by the method. Most methods have helped some cerebral palsied children, but every method has failings. Some cerebral palsied children improve without treatment. No scientific evidence available today demonstrates that any *one* method of treatment is superior to all other methods. No currently employed system of treating cerebral palsied children has been adequately tested through carefully controlled studies.

Depending on where she is employed a therapist might encounter any of several systems of treating cerebral palsied children. None of these systems can be learned from reading a book. They all require both study with someone who is trained in the system and supervised practice with cerebral palsied children. There is no better way to prepare for the varying philosophies and procedures which the therapist might be expected to know and use than to develop an understanding of the fundamental neurophysiological and psychological concepts on which all diagnostic and therapeutic procedures are based.

> 45   After reading Hellebrandt (*81*: 9-14), Ayres (*6*: 302-10), Semans (*161*: 99-110), Curran (*33*: 80-87), Shelton (*163*: 855-59), Perlstein in (*34*), and Denhoff (*43*), and Robinault make a list of the principles on which procedures for treatment cerebral palsied children should be based. As you study each of the following systems of therapy determine to what extent the system observes the basic principles. (The Curran chart is a good starting point.)

System of Therapy Developed by Winthrop Phelps

One of the earliest systematic programs for the treatment of children with cerebral palsy was that developed by Phelps (*141*: 3-5), (*144*: 1004-12), (*145*: 136-38), Egel (*49*), and St. James (*170*: 102-106). In this method the treatment of individual muscles is stressed, hence, the therapist must learn to identify both the disordered muscles and those muscles which are functioning normally. After the physician's examination establishes the neurological diagnosis, a detailed muscle examination is made by a trainer who is usually a physical therapist. Several types of muscle condition might be recognized. A normal muscle is one which is capable of contracting to the desired degree of tenseness and to relax when its antagonist contracts. A spastic muscle is hyperirritable and reacts to stretching by contraction which interferes with motion. A flaccid muscle, also called a *zero cerebral,* does not have the power to contract voluntarily. In athetosis, muscles contract involuntarily and thus interfere with voluntary motion. Also to be noted is the presence of pathological overflow. In normal individuals, overflow often occurs when a person protrudes his tongue while trying to thread a needle. In the cerebral palsied, a stretch reflex may spread from the point where it was originally stimulated to produce stretch reflexes in other parts of the body. Athetosis is frequently seen to spread from motions around one joint to include motions around many joints. Muscles are also graded according to the amount of power they possess.

After the muscle examination has determined the condition of important muscles, the child is enrolled in a treatment program which consists of fifteen modalities. Modalities are phases of treatment which have been developed for cerebral palsied conditions. The first modality, *massage,* is used to increase the power and tone of weak muscles by improving the circulation and nutrition of indivdual muscles. Actually this modality is not often used in the treatment of cerebral palsy. Treatment is more likely to begin with the second modality, *passive motion.* The basic assumption behind this modality is that before a cerebral palsied child can correct an abnormal motion he must be shown how to make the motion by the therapist. The latter moves the appropriate parts of the cerebral palsied person's body through the motion with no voluntary effort on the part of the child. Passive motion is followed by *active assisted motion* in which the therapist, with a small degree of effort from the child, moves the body parts through the desired pattern of movement. In the next modality, *active motion,* the child voluntarily carries out the desired motion with no help from the therapist other than counting to regulate the range and speed of the motion. Obviously the child capable of controlled, active motion has attained a high degree of neuromotor coordination. This modality, therefore, represents an advanced stage of treatment. It is achieved by a progression from the starting points of massage and passive motion through active, assisted motion.

There are several other modalities which have special applications. *Resisted motion,* a modality in which the therapist manually applies a force opposing the child's movement, is used in the final stages of treatment to build up the power of individual muscles or muscle groups. *Conditioned motion* is the name given to a modality in which a specific rhyme is sung to the child for each motion taught during the passive and active assisted-motion stages of treatment. Through conditioning, the child will automatically carry out the motion which is associated with the rhyme when the therapist sings the rhyme as a stimulus. A rhyme and melody have been standardized for each motion.

Still another modality, *automatic or confused motion,* is used for flaccid muscles which might be activated by an overflow of impulses from a resisted motion of another part of the body. It is felt that individuals differ in the pattern of confused motions of which they are capable. A resistance which produces an automatic action in one individual might not work on other individuals. However, by careful exploration, the therapist can usually find a confusion pattern which will result in the desired muscle response. Confusion actions are used to build up strength in flaccid muscles. However, regardless of how strong the flaccid muscle becomes, it can never contract independently of the total pattern of resistance and confused motion.

Combined motions constitute an advanced modality which must be taught to all types of cerebral palsied children. Since most useful acts require movement at several joints, the ability to perform active motions around one joint will not be adequate for learning self-help skills. The combined-motion modality teaches the child to carry out motions involving combinations of movements at two joints. For example, the child would be taught the finger flexion with wrist extension which is basic for grasping.

In another modality, *rest,* body braces, special chairs and tables, corsets, and other devices are used to control the motions which use up much of the cerebral palsied individual's energy. In addition an effort is made to see that the cerebral palsied child has optimal sleep and diet habits. A systematic program of *relaxation* is carried out to train the child to produce physiologic relaxation of tense muscles. By teaching the child to recognize the sensations of tightness and looseness of muscles, this modality aims to reduce the tension and involuntary motion which interferes with purposeful movement.

A modality known as *motion from the relaxed position* is used primarily with athetoids. Ability to *balance* is essential for such motor activities as sitting, kneeling, crawling, standing, and walking; so, balance training is an important modality in the treatment of cerebral palsied children. *Reciprocation* is an important modality for all cerebral palsied cases and is employed in conjunction with other modalities from the beginning of treatment. The passive, active-assisted, and active motions employed are often reciprocal in nature. An important modality for upper-extremity training is *reach and grasp*. This modality is one of the last steps in the treatment for all cerebral palsied patients and requires the learning of combined motions involving two or more joints in one extremity. The final modality is known as *skills*. This final step in the treatment of the cerebral palsied child stresses feeding, dressing, toilet care, writing, and typing.

Specific techniques have been developed for each of the modalities. Special equipment such as braces, twisters, stabilizers, relaxation chairs, standing tables, and other devices are employed in carrying out the modalities.

46   Speech is regarded by Phelps as a fifth extremity along with arms and legs. Which modalities are applicable to speech therapy and how are they employed? See Westlake (188), (189), Cass (21), Gratke (70), and Rutherford (155.)

System of Therapy Developed by Karl and Berta Bobath

The Bobaths (14: 146-53), (15: 4-10), (16: 146-53), (17: 88-89) note that there are four levels of integration of motor function: a spinal level, a brain-stem level, a midbrain level, and a cortical level. With maturation of the central nervous system there is a gradual shift from spinal-level integration to integration at the cortical level as the lower-level reflexes are brought under the inhibitory control of higher centers.

In cerebral palsy (according to these authors) the damaged brain is unable to bring the lower levels under the inhibitory control of the higher levels. The child's motor behavior is dominated by spinal and brain-stem reflexes which interfere with the development of midbrain and cortically integrated patterns. The flexor withdrawal reflex, the extensor thrust, and the crossed extension reflex—all of which are integrated at the spinal level—are often seen in cerebral palsied children. Cerebral palsied children also show the asymmetrical tonic neck reflex, symmetrical tonic neck reflex, tonic labyrinthine reflex, the positive and negative supporting reactions, and the associated reactions which are integrated in the brain stem. Persistence of tonic reflexes produces a strong increase in muscle tone and stereotyped postures.

Many cerebral palsied children have difficulty in developing the midbrain-integrated righting reflexes which are important for rolling, sitting, crawling, and standing. Also absent or poorly developed in many cerebral palsied children are the equilibrium reactions which are integrated by the basal ganglia, cerebellum, and cortex. These reactions represent the highest level of reflexive maturation. While lower-level reflexes disappear as the normal central nervous system matures, the equilibrium reactions persist throughout life. In cerebral palsied children the lower-level reflexes persist and the equilibrium reflexes fail to develop.

From the time of birth we are bombarded by sensory stimulation. The normal nervous system can respond with a great variety of appropriate motor reactions. The cerebral palsied child, however, is incapable of varied and selective motor responses. His motor activity is limited to the persistent spinal and tonic reflexes and perhaps to some primitive righting reactions. In the Bobaths' view this causes the afferent inflow to be shunted into the few synaptic channels which have been established by the dominance of the spinal, brain-stem, and midbrain reflexes. In the milder cases, i.e., those in whom the spinal, brain-stem and midbrain reflexes are not so strong, the abnormal reflex activity is modified by voluntary compensatory activity, though the underlying reflex synergies can still be seen. Some of the righting and equilibrium reactions which are integrated at higher levels may be present, but they are not fully developed and their harmonious interplay is always lacking.

Shunting accounts for the stereotyped motor activities of the child who has persistent spinal and tonic reflexes. Muscles which are contracted and those which are elongated send afferent impulses to the central nervous system which uses this sensory information to determine which muscles should be activated and which should be inhibited. The afferent inflow from contracted and elongated muscles makes it likely that the C.N.S. will stimulate the elongated muscle to contract and will inhibit the contracted muscle. The *law of shunting* states that at any moment the C.N.S. mirrors the state of the body musculature. To put it another way, excitation from the central nervous system is likely to flow into the stretched muscle. When tonic reflexes persist, certain muscles are contracted much of the time while certain other muscles are usually elongated, hence, the central nervous system is "set" to produce a stereotyped distribution of excitatory and inhibitory impulses.

Shunting also provides a mechanism for inhibiting the tonic reflex activity and for facilitating righting and equilibrium reactions. By positioning the child in such a way as to elongate the muscles which were contracted and to contract those muscles which were elongated, it is possible to create a different pattern of sensory inflow to the C.N.S. In this way new neural circuits are opened. Inhibition of tonic reflex activity through the use of *reflex inhibiting postures* (*RIPS*) produces a more normal state of muscle tone, making it possible to *facilitate* movement following normal developmental sequences. Initial *RIPS* attempt to achieve a complete reversal of the muscle picture associated with the abnormal posture. For example, a child with a predominantly extensor pattern would be flexed at all major joints. As treatment progresses, many postures are used in an effort to weaken the tonic reflexes and to open up a variety of neural circuits. Permanent inhibition of the tonic reflexes is achieved by developing righting and equilibrium reactions.

In using this method of treatment with a child it is necessary that the physical, speech, and occupational therapists work closely together. Each must be trained to recognize the reflex patterns which are integrated at the various levels of the C.N.S. Each must know the normal sequences of reflex development and know how to inhibit persistent tonic reflexes. Physical therapists must know how to facilitate righting and equilibrium reactions in their proper developmental sequences. The speech therapist must learn how to dissociate the movements of breathing and speech from movements of other parts of the body, how to facilitate voice production and babbling, and how to use RIPS when developing articulatory movements.

> **47** How are the concepts of inhibition of persistent tonic reflexes and facilitation of movement applicable to speech therapy for the cerebral palsied? See Crickmay (29), Marland (114: 111-19), Mysak (122) and (123: 221-30).

System of Therapy Developed by Margaret Rood

Techniques for treating neuromuscular dysfunction which are based on the activation, facilitation, and inhibition of muscle action through stimulation of sensory receptors have been described by Rood (152: 444-50), (153: 525-27), (119). She notes that a child must have developed the lower-level reflexes before he can develop higher-level voluntary control. Normally reflexes and motor skills follow definite developmental sequences. In the cerebral palsied child, motor patterns do not appear in their proper sequence because the sensory-motor pathways are not intact. Impulses are not transmitted across synapses because the threshold is too high. A child must first feel a pattern of muscle contraction before he can reproduce it. Asking a child who has never felt the pattern of muscle contraction to perform an action voluntarily does not assist him in getting the feel of the movement. Passively moving a limb through its range of motion does not enable the patient to experience the proper stimulation associated with the movement. By appropriate activation of sensory receptors, the synaptic thresholds can be lowered, thus facilitating action and making it possible to develop patterns of movements in their proper developmental sequences.

Muscle function, according to Miss Rood, is of two types. One function is for maintaining posture and heavy work. The other is for range and speed, i.e., light work. The type of sensory stimulation to be employed depends on the function of the muscle which is to be activated. Some muscles are designed for both light and heavy work.

Exteroceptors located in the skin are primitive sense organs. They

have fine fibers, are slow to react, and have a long after-discharge. Because these skin receptors are diffusely distributed, their stimulation
evokes whole, rather than selective, reaction patterns. Stimulation of
the skin receptors causes reciprocal innervation in which an agonist is
activated while the antagonist is inhibited. Since the sensory end organs
have superficial locations, they may be stimulated by brushing. Rapid
brushing (5 strokes per second) for about thirty seconds results in activation. Slow, rhythmic, continuous brushing for about three minutes
produces inhibition.

Proprioceptors are located in muscles, tendons, joints, and bones
and are activated by position, stretch, and pressure. The position of
the head influences the kind and locus of muscle tone through the labyrinthine reflexes. Stretching of a muscle stimulates the muscle spindle
which triggers a quick-acting, two-neuron reflex. Muscle-spindle function is important for primitive, heavy-work patterns. The Golgi end
organs, which are located in tendons, are inhibitory and stop the
stretch action in the muscle. Pressures applied to pressure receptors in
the fascia between layers of muscles, to the insertion of a muscle on
a bone, and to the bone itself give rise to proprioceptive impulses.

On the surface of the body, areas have been identified which are
supplied by nerve fibers from an afferent spinal root. These areas, which
are called *skin fields* or *dermatomes,* are sensory representations for
muscles innervated through a corresponding segment of the spinal cord.
A myotome includes all the muscles supplied by one section of the
cord. Stimulation of a dermatome by stroking or brushing, for example,
activates the muscle or muscles with which the dermatome is associated.

48   Review the discussions and illustrations of dermatomes in the Ciba
      volume on the nervous system (*125*), Gardner (*61*), Fulton (*60*), Sherring-
      ton (*164*). Identify the skin areas associated with breathing, sucking,
      and swallowing.

Muscles may also be activated by stroking the skin area over the
belly of the muscle or the area over its insertion. Brushing activates
light-work muscles. It facilitates but does not activate heavy-work
muscles. Heavy-work muscles are activated by stretching and pressure.
Brushing, according to Miss Rood, produces long-lasting effects.
Pressures are effective only during the time of their application. Thermal stimuli, ice and warm towels, are also effective. Application of ice
affects the fine fibers which are involved in primitive, protective types
of motor patterns. Warm applications bring in fibers associated with
more specific effects. Stimulation must follow a sequence. Brushing or

stroking comes first to facilitate muscle action. Then, for heavy-work muscles, pressures are applied to the belly of the muscle, then to the insertion of the muscle, and finally reinforced with bone pressures. If a muscle can't be stimulated to work reflexly, brushing should be followed by icing. When more discriminating functions are desired, warm applications should precede brushing.

Two types of functions are identified: skeletal functions and vital functions. For each, motor activities must be developed in their normal developmental sequences. The withdrawal reflex must be established first because it is the foundation from which other skeletal functions develop. By applying appropriate stimuli to facilitate, activate, or inhibit a selected muscle or group of muscles, children are helped to progress from withdrawal through rolling, creeping, and standing to walking. Techniques for developing upper-extremity skeletal functions have also been worked out.

The developmental sequence of vital functions also follows a progression from primitive to skilled. The progression, as described by Rood, is respiration, crying, sucking, swallowing fluids, speech, chewing, and swallowing solids. Appropriate sensory stimuli are proposed for the facilitation and activation and inhibition of muscles involved in each of these vital functions.

To use these techniques intelligently, a therapist must know the location and action of muscles, the dermatomes of pertinent muscles, developmental sequences of skeletal and vital functions, and the muscles responsible for producing each motor pattern. After acquiring this basic information, the therapist must learn to analyze the various patterns to determine what stimulation is necessary. Therapists should resist the temptation to use brushes, ice, and pressures without first learning where, when, and how to employ these stimuli.

> 49   How are the techniques of inhibition and facilitation described by Miss Rood applicable in helping the cerebral palsied child develop adequate breathing, sucking, chewing, swallowing, and speech patterns? See Rood (*151*: 220-24), Moyer and Davis, eds. (*119*), Mysak (*122*).

System of Therapy Developed by Herman Kabat and Margaret Knott

The theories and techniques of neuromuscular re-education developed by Kabat (*93*), (*94*: 190-204), (*95*: 23-24) have been elaborated by Knott (*101*: 1-3) and Knott and Voss (*102*). The rationale for this technique notes that normal actions are produced by synergistic contractions of a group of muscles rather than by single joint movements.

Since a single muscle or an isolated motion is practically never used in the performance of voluntary activities, treatment procedures concentrating on isolated muscles or isolated motions are regarded by Kabat as being ineffective and unsound. Modalities such as passive motion and assistive motion activate only a small percentage of the motor units of a muscle. Such treatment affords little opportunity for motor learning.

A more effective method of neuromuscular training would attempt to achieve maximal activation of the neuromuscular mechanism with each voluntary effort. This technique attempts to increase the excitation in the central nervous system by applying strong resistance to mass-movement patterns. Resisted movement requires maximum effort on the part of the patient with a resultant increase in the number of motor units activated and the activation of dormant neurons.

Analysis of the mass-movement patterns shows that they are predominantly diagonal-spiral patterns. Ready examples of such movements may be seen in the body rotation which accompanies a serve in tennis or in rolling to the right side from the supine position. It is pointed out that when normals attempt to get power and endurance in motions, they employ diagonal patterns. A lumberjack, for example, does not use straight flexion-extension movements of the trunk and arms when cutting a tree with an ax. Rotation of the trunk and arms can easily be seen in this action.

These techniques have become known as *proprioceptive neuromuscular facilitation techniques* because of their emphasis on proprioceptor stimulation. Resistance to a movement is achieved by the therapist who applies counterpressure against the surface toward which the motion is made. In a synergistic movement the various components of a pattern respond in a definite sequence, hence, attention must be given to the proper timing of the application of resistance. Attention is also given to starting position and range of motion in teaching patterns to cerebral palsied children. Care must be exercised to avoid applying resistance simultaneously to the agonist and antagonist directions.

Mass-movement patterns are reinforced through repeated contractions, slow reversal, and rhythmic stabilization. *Repeated contractions* are used to develop power and endurance in single direction of movement. In this technique, the patient attempts a voluntary contraction in that part of the range of motion which is most easy for him to manage. This voluntary contraction is followed by an isometric contraction against resistence. Without relaxing the muscle the patient repeats a number of isotonic contractions against maximum resistance. The *slow-reversal method* of reinforcement employs isotonic contractions against maximum resistance. First, maximum isotonic contraction of the antagonist is elicited and then without relaxation the patient reverses to a maximum isotonic contraction of the agonist. This procedure is carried out several times at different points in the range of motion.

Rhythmic stabilization employs isometric contractions. The patient attempts to hold a joint rigid against resistance which the therapist applies first to one antagonist and then to the other. These reinforcement techniques are not equally applicable to all types of cerebral palsy. Repeated contractions may be employed effectively with spastics, ataxics, and athetoids. The slow-reversal reinforcement procedure is effective with ataxics and athetoids, but these types of cerebral palsied individuals do not learn to perform rhythmic-stabilization activities. This technique is more effective with spastics.

To employ these proprioceptive neuromuscular facilitation techniques in the treatment of cerebral palsied patients, a therapist would need to know the mass-movement patterns and their components. It would be essential to know how, where, and when to apply maximum resistance. The therapist must be skilled in employing the appropriate techniques for reinforcing the mass-movement patterns.

50 In what ways can a speech therapist use such techniques as strong resistance to mass-movement patterns and reinforcement of mass-movement patterns through repeated contractions, slow reversal, and rhythmic stabilization in the treatment of cerebral palsied children? See Lefevre (*104*: 61-65) and Hoberman (*82*: 111-23).

System of Therapy Developed by Temple Fay

A method of treating cerebral palsied children by eliciting primitive movement patterns has been described by Fay (*53*: 200-203), (*54*: 327-34), (*55*: 644-52), (*56*: 347-52).

From studies of the comparative anatomy of the vertebrate nervous system, Fay notes that many features of the nervous system have persisted throughout the evolution of vertebrates. For example, the twelve pairs of cranial nerves are found in all vertebrates and the basic functions of each pair has remained the same throughout evolution. Further, similarity in the bony structure of the extremities is also apparent throughout the evolution of vertebrates.

Analysis of the movement patterns of fish, amphibians, reptiles, and newborn human infants reveals a striking similarity in the patterns. Postural reflexes, reactions of defense, tonic neck reflexes and pattern movements are motor activities integrated by the phylogenetically older brain. These patterns are still latent in man and may be seen in analyzing the ontogenetic recapitulation of phylogenetic development. *Homolateral* movements in which the upper and lower extremity on the same side move together are characteristic of the amphibian level of development. *Homologous* movements in which both upper extremities move together and both lower extremities move together are found in the amphibian as well as in higher levels. The next higher type of movement is the *crossed-diagonal pattern* which appears in reptiles. In this pattern the right front leg and the left rear leg would function together as would the left front leg and the right rear leg. This pattern is seen in the trotting gait of horses. In man the persistence of this pattern may be seen in the contralateral movements of arms and legs in walking.

While the cerebral palsied child may be unable to produce voluntary movement, he often retains many spontaneous reflex-pattern movements. Homolateral movements may be elicited by turning the head from side to side with the child in a prone position. Passive movement of the extremities in time with the alternation of head position induces the amphibian crawling-movement pattern. Repetition of this pattern leads to the reptilian or crossed-diagonal pattern. At this level of treatment, contralateral movements of the extremities are timed with alternations of head position.

Therapy attempts to organize and coordinate lower-level reflex activities with the undamaged portions of higher cortical centers. In this way the basic automatic reflexes are elicited (in the order of their phylogenetic appearance) to develop muscles, to relax antagonists, and to produce better coordination of muscle tone. Reflexes are organized to produce a sequence of homolateral crawling patterns, contralateral crawling patterns, quadrupedal creeping, and upright locomotion.

In addition to eliciting the patterned movements of the type just described, this therapy also stimulates appropriate defense reactions to improve the function of various muscle groups. For example the withdrawal pattern may be elicited to help a child develop control of a lower extremity. Many reflex responses have been identified which involve activation of muscles through lower-level integrative mechanisms when cortical function is defective. Fay has described many procedures for "unlocking" reflexes, i.e., using specific stimuli to break up unwanted reflex patterns.

To employ this method, which is often referred to as *patterning,* a therapist should know the sequences of both the phylogenetic and ontogenetic developmental patterns. Understanding of procedures for reproducing the patterns and for breaking up unwanted patterns is essential.

51   There are many other approaches to treating cerebral palsied children.
      What are the emphases of Deaver (*37*), (*38:* 363-67), Gillette (*65:* 31-34),
      (*66:* 56-59), and Collis (*25:* 139-44), (*26*)? What systems of therapy have
      influenced the approaches of Palmer (*127:* 193-202), (*128:* 514), (*129:*
      3-6), Kastein (*97:* 17-20), (*98:* 4-19), and Mecham (*115*) to speech and
      language training for cerebral palsied children?

Which system of therapy for cerebral palsied children is best? No one knows and the problems of research design are so difficult that it will be a long time before satisfactorily controlled evaluative studies can be conducted. A new therapist must reconcile himself to learning techniques of the system used by other members of the team or group. It is widely recognized today that merely having physical, occupational, and speech therapists on the staff does not assure the child of an effective program. Only when the efforts of therapists are fully integrated can effective treatment for cerebral palsied children be provided. At one time physical therapists, occupational therapists, and speech therapists saw sharp distinctions among their functions. The physical therapist was concerned primarily with developing walking skills, the occupational therapist with the self-help skills, and the speech therapist with developing speech and language functions. There was little overlapping among their various activities.

With the growing awareness of the unitary character of the human-reaction mechanism, boundaries between therapies have broken down. Knowledge that the nervous system as a whole contributes to every motor act makes it unsound for the speech therapist to work on tongue or jaw movements without consideration of the presence of flexor or extensor tone in other parts of the body. No longer can the occupational therapist work on hand skills without attention to such factors as posture and its effect on muscle tone in the upper extremities. Our awareness that part functions individuate from total postural and movement patterns lead all therapists to employ procedures which influence the organism as a whole.

Unfortunately, many therapists are not familiar with the physiology of motor learning, the psychological bases of learning, and therapeutic techniques by which physiological and psychological principles can be employed in habilitating the cerebral palsied child. Agencies concerned with treating cerebral palsied children should make provisions for a continuous program of in-service training for therapists and other professional personnnel. Therapists should attend an appropriate short course designed to teach one of the treatment approaches, keep up with professional literature, and attend pertinent professional meetings.

Each therapist should accept the individual responsibility of learning as much as possible about cerebral palsy and its treatment.

> 52   What short-term training programs are offered in cerebral palsy and what financial aid is available? Write to the National Society for Crippled Children and Adults and to United Cerebral Palsy for information.

BRACING AND SPECIAL EQUIPMENT IN THE TREATMENT OF CEREBRAL PALSY[1]

Seeing a cerebral palsied child wearing heavy braces which restrict his motions is often a distressing sight for a beginning therapist or teacher. Similarly, to one unacquainted with their purpose, special chairs, tables, and other equipment may appear unattractive and even foreboding. The need for bracing and for special equipment arises from the child's disturbed neuromuscular function. Since his muscles cannot stabilize joints, he has difficulty maintaining desirable postures without outside help. Overly strong muscles can also produce deformities unless their power is counteracted.

There are differences of opinion about the value of bracing and other types of special equipment in the treatment of cerebral palsy. Some physicians regard bracing as one of the most valuable adjuncts in the treatment program. There are others who feel that bracing is contraindicated with cerebral palsied patients. In some clinics bracing and special equipment are used extensively; in others only occasional use

> 53   To brace or not to brace—that is the questioned raised by specialists in treating cerebral palsy. Research evidence is lacking, but clinical opinions on each side have some strong arguments. Compare Deaver (38: 363-67) and Collis (25: 139-44).

will be made of these treatment adjuncts. Bracing will not be used at all in some treatment centers. Therapists should understand the philosophy behind each approach.

Bracing

In the treatment of cerebral palsy, bracing is used to provide needed support, to control involuntary movements, to prevent or correct deformities—or for some combination of these objectives. One of the

---

[1]For photographs and drawings of braces and special equipment see the publications of The National Society for Crippled Children and Adults, *Foundations for Walking, An Exhibit of Therapeutic Equipment for Cerebral Palsied Children* and *A Manual of Cerebral Palsy Equipment*.

most commonly used braces is the *short leg brace* which is employed to control foot position, to prevent heel-cord tightening, and to stabilize ankle motion. A short leg brace consists of a bar which is attached at its upper end to a calf cuff. See Fig. 5. The lower end is attached to a caliper box which is built into the bottom of a shoe. The angle of the foot in relation to the leg, that is, the amount of dorsiflexion or plantar flexion, may be adjusted by bending the bar with brace irons or through an adjustable stop on the caliper box. Short leg braces may be worn only during the day, but since spasticity is present even while the child sleeps, bracing may be continued during the night. Mild spastics might wear a night brace only.

When it is necessary to provide support for control at the knee, a *long leg brace* is used. This brace consists of a thigh cuff to which are attached two long bars, one on the inside and the other on the outside, which extend downward to the shoe. At the knee, a knee pad attached to the bars helps hold the leg in position. The bars are jointed at the knee to allow for flexion and extension movements. A locking arrangement at the knee will hold the leg in a desired angle of extension.

When support or control of the hip joint is necessary, the outside bar on the long leg brace is continued upward and attached to a pelvic band. The bar is jointed at the hip and provided with a locking arrangement. Sometimes it is necessary for a child to wear braces on

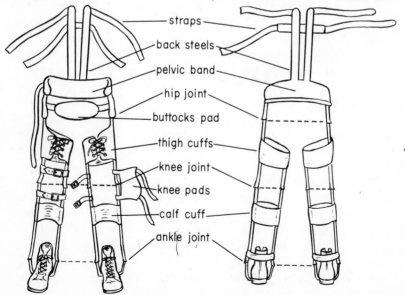

straps
back steels
pelvic band
hip joint
buttocks pad
thigh cuffs
knee joint
knee pads
calf cuff
ankle joint

Figure 5. Parts of a Body Brace Used in the Treatment of Cerebral Palsy.

both legs. For children with poor trunk stability because of weakness
or involuntary motion of trunk and arm muscles, the brace is extended
upward from the pelvic band by adding back steels and shoulder straps.
Sometimes a corset is added to provide additional trunk support.

> **54**   Would bracing be done in the same way for the spastic, athetoid, ataxic,
>   rigidity, and tremor types of cerebral palsy? See Koven (*103*: 4-7), Phelps
>   (*142*: 1-3), (*143*), and Hastings (*78*: 1-6).

Weighted shoes may be used to produce a lower center of gravity for
the cerebral palsied child who is beginning to walk. For the beginning
walker, shoes with platform soles (sometimes called *duck shoes*), which
provide a greater area of contact with the floor, may be used to provide more stability. To counteract internal or external rotation of the
legs, *twisters* are used. These may be straps which are attached to a
corset and wrapped around the leg. The lower end of the strap is
attached to the shoe. A newer model consists of a metal coil attached
at the upper end to a pelvic band and at the lower end to a shoe.
Torquing of the coil pulls the leg in the desired position.

Bracing of the upper extremities is less common than bracing for
the lower extremities and the trunk. In part this is because support of
the upper extremities is not needed for maintaining an erect position.
Bracing to correct or prevent deformities of the upper extremity is very
difficult. Most physicians consider it impractical to brace the shoulder
and elbow joints in cerebral palsy. Bracing of spastic hands to counteract flexion deformities will be the most common type of upper-extremity bracing the therapist will encounter. Therapists often request some
kind of head support for cerebral palsied children who have weak or
flaccid neck muscles. Since many of these children have poor arm and
hand control, a rigid brace which rests on the shoulders and holds the
chin up can be dangerous. If an unattended child's chin should become
caught over the top of the brace, strangulation might occur. Sometimes an extension from the back brace is attached to a helmet to control head position.

Braces are used only after a careful evaluation of the child's muscle
status, posture, and deformities. Braces must be carefully designed
and constructed to restrict unwanted motions, to allow desired motions,
to prevent deformities, and to provide necessary support. When bracing is used with a child, the therapist should become familiar with its
objectives. Ordinarily the physical therapist will be primarily responsible for teaching the child to use his braces. The other therapists and
teachers should know how to lock and unlock a child's braces and

how to tell if they have been put on the child properly. To put a child in a long leg brace or full body brace requires ten to fifteen minutes. Problems sometimes arise when one therapist wants the child to be unbraced during treatment while the other therapists want him to be braced. If there are good reasons for wanting to treat the child without his braces, these should be discussed with other staff members and supervisors so that a satisfactory treatment schedule can be arranged.

> 55   Therapists and parents must guard against straining their back and abdominal muscles when lifting cerebral palsied children. What are the proper methods of lifting a child from the floor and from a chair? See Shriner (166) and Moorehouse (118).

Special Equipment

Because the cerebral palsied child is unable to follow normal developmental sequences at a normal rate, special equipment is used to assist him in sitting, standing, and walking.

One of the most commonly used items of special equipment is the relaxation chair. For children who go into a flexed position with the head dropped forward, shoulders slumped, and the upper part of the body pressing down on the abdominal areas, visual contact with the environment is limited, hand and arm function is restricted, and the development of an adequate speech-breathing pattern is often difficult. A chair with an adjustable seat and back can be tilted backward to help the child maintain a better position of his head and trunk. By decreasing the angle at which the seat is attached to the back of the chair (sometimes referred to as *jackknifing*), it is possible to maintain the child in a partially flexed position and thus counteract the strong extensor thrusts seen in some children. Since relaxation chairs improve the child's position for hand function and feeding training, they are commonly used in occupational therapy activities. More general use should be considered for any child whose poor sitting posture interferes with the development of adequate speech-breathing patterns and visual exploration of his environment.

> 56   At what age should the use of a relaxation chair be considered and what factors should be considered in designing and fitting a chair for a cerebral palsied child? See Perlstein (139) and Shriner (166).

The normal child, during the second half of his first year, spends a great deal of time pulling himself to a standing position and standing with support in preparation for walking. Through these activities, he develops strength, balance, and other reflexes. To provide similar opportunities for cerebral palsied children, a standing table is used. Such a table consists of a long rectangular box which is set upright on a firm base. When the child is standing in this box or chimney, the upper rim should reach to just below his armpits. The box should fit snugly enough to provide support but should allow enough movement to help the child develop balance reflexes. A divider may be used to prevent scissoring of the legs. A tray or table which is attached to the chimney holds toys, books, and other materials for the child. Several chimneys may be attached to one large table, thus giving the child opportunities to stand and play in company with other children.

> 57   What factors must be considered in determining when a child should
>   use a standing table, for how long he should stand at a time, and how
>   the standing table should be adjusted for him? See Perlstein et al. (139)
>   and Shriner (166).

Among the other items of special equipment used in the treatment of cerebral palsy are stabilizers which are used to develop standing balance by gradually decreasing the level at which the child is supported, parallel bars for developing reciprocal hand and leg motions, weighted and tripod canes, crutches, and other devices to assist in developing walking skills. While the responsibility for using these devices will usually be that of the physical therapist, the speech therapist should know with what special equipment each child is working and should discuss with the physical therapist ways of relating speech and language activities to the physical therapy program. For example, it might be possible for the physical therapist to work on the child's speech-breathing pattern while he is standing in a stabilizer.

What special equipment might be used with the cerebral palsied children we met in Chapter I? Perhaps Carl Pednok should have a short leg brace to counteract the tight right heel cord which causes him to walk on the toes of his right foot. However, a regularly used night brace might keep the heel cord stretched sufficiently. Would you want to consider the use of a relaxation chair with Clayton Penths? Is Clayton ready for a standing table? What kind of bracing do you think a physician might order for Charleen Pimskon? Is she ready for any other special equipment? Analyze the bracing and equipment needs of each child as fully as you can from the information given about them in Chapter I.   ♪♪♪

THERE ARE CONTRIBUTIONS TO BE MADE BY ALL THE THERAPISTS AND teachers to a cerebral palsied child's language and speech development, but the major responsibility for this program usually is that of the speech and hearing therapist. In this section we will present some models which can serve as guides for developing language and speech in the young child, can provide a basis for diagnosing language and speech problems in the older child, and can give direction to the planing of therapy.

A number of definitions of language have been formulated and models of language function have been developed. Confused thinking and ineffective treatment sometimes arises from a failure to distinguish between language, speech, and the processes by which speech is produced. Unless meaningful distinctions are made, the therapist some-

6

language and speech
problems: diagnosis

times works on speech problems when the basic difficulties are language deficits. Because a frame of reference for diagnosing was not used, therapy has sometimes been directed toward one of the processes by which speech is produced when more basic defects exist in other processes.

58 After studying the recent theoretical models of Osgood (126), Wepman *et al.* (184: 323-32), and Kirk and McCarthy (100: 399-412) identify their similarities and describe them. Where possible reconcile the differences.

Before starting to treat a cerebral palsied child, the speech and hearing therapist should attempt to answer three questions: *What is the nature of the child's language and speech difficulty? What are the causes of the difficulty? What can be done to improve the child's language and speech skills?* Only after tenable, if tentative, answers to these three questions have been formulated is the therapist ready to begin treating the child. To be adequate, an evaluation must identify specific processes or functions to be treated and suggest specific therapeutic techniques.

FOUNDATIONS OF LANGUAGE DEVELOPMENT

Experiences are essential to the development of language. As the human organism interacts with its environment, experience comes naturally. The passage of time affords ever increasing opportunities for experience to accrue. The quality of the experience is determined by the capabilities of the organism, the characteristics of the environment, and the amount of time the organism has had to interact with its environment. Experiences occur first as awarenesses of environmental stimuli, i.e., sensations. With increasing maturity the child learns to detect differences between stimuli and these discriminations assist him in giving meaning to his sensations. Perceptions occur when sensations are differentiated and become meaningful. Concepts, the core material of which language is constructed, are perceptions which have been generalized and classified.

There are several modalities through which language is utilized: listening, speaking, gesturing, thinking, reading, and writing. Not only do these modalities use language, but they also create language. As one reads, listens, thinks, or talks, he develops new concepts and thus adds to his language. This relationship is suggested by the double-headed arrow pointing from language to the modality and from the modality back to language in Fig. 6.

Structural and Functional Integrity

The base of the foundation on which our language structure develops is structural and functional integrity or the ability to compensate for deficits. Structural anomalies might affect the development of one modality without affecting other modalities or the development of language itself. For example, paralysis of the tongue would affect speech production but not necessarily interfere with language development or the development of other modalities for language use. Neuromuscular problems in the upper extremities might interfere with writing but not necessarily with the development of language or some of the other modalities for language use.

Of particular importance to the development of language is the integrity of the reaction mechanism. For experiences to occur, the organism and the environment must act on each other. Action on the part of the organism involves assuming postures and carrying out movements. Moving and posturing occur as the result of patterns

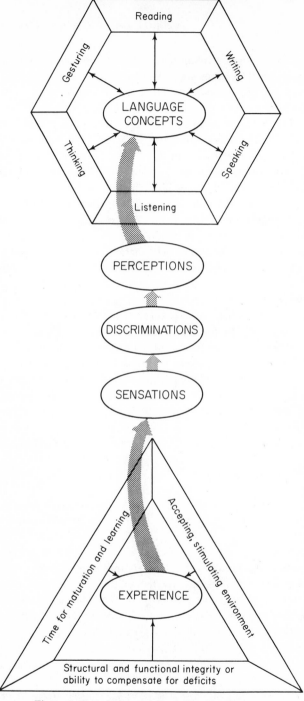

Figure 6. Foundations of Language Development.

of muscle activation and inhibition. When the effector system functions normally, the child creates for himself countless opportunities to add to his experiential background. These opportunities tend to decrease in number as the motor disabilities of a child increase.

The sensorium must be responsive to environmental stimuli in order for sensations, the most primitive level of experiencing, to occur. Further, the sensory system must be able to feed back information about the manner in which the motor or effector portion of the reaction mechanism is functioning. The common sensory malfunctionings of cerebral palsied children have been described in Chapter IV.

Neural impulses from the sensory end organs must be interpreted in the central nervous system; in addition, they must also be integrated with other incoming stimuli and with data stored from previous stimulations. For reflexive motor acts, as when a child quickly withdraws his hand from a hot stove, the process of symbolization is not involved. When the child avoids touching a stove because his mother tells him it is hot and has learned from previous experience that hot things are painful, the ability to formulate and manipulate symbols assists his nervous system in interpreting and integrating incoming information. Symbol formulation is essential to concept development. The neurophysiology of symbol formulation and manipulation is not completely understood, but it is known that this ability can be lost or disturbed by brain damage such as that associated with strokes, penetrating wounds of the brain, or other cerebral traumas. It is also possible that because of developmental or acquired brain defects, children may find it difficult or impossible to develop language. These deficits may be specific to a modality such as reading or speaking, or the deficits may be

59   There is continuing professional debate about the existence of congenital aphasia, but as Wood (191) points out, the arguments are largely semantic. How would aphasia be diagnosed in a child? See Wood (191), West (185), Myklebust (120).

more general. The ability to interpret and integrate stimuli for the formulation of symbols is also related to the general intellectual level of the child. Limited intellectual potential imposes limitations on language development. However, it is possible for a child with a language disability to have good intellectual potential.

Environment

The second portion of the foundation for our language structure is the environment. In a very real sense, we cannot speak of the environment as being separate from the organism, for the organism is an integral part of its environment. The environment changes as the child enters it and continues to change with his changes in posture or movement. Suppose that a child visually explores an environment which consists of a block on a table. As soon as he reaches for the block, the environment which he sees now includes his moving hand. Or let us suppose that a child is in auditory contact with an environment composed of usual sounds created in a home. When he vocalizes, this auditory environment changes immediately as the sound produced by him becomes a part of the environmental stimuli of which he is aware. A normal child constantly changes his visual environment by looking in different directions, by using his extremities to manipulate objects within his field of vision, and later by moving his entire body to different parts of his environment. Similarly he changes his auditory environment by remaining quiet or by crying, cooing, babbling, and so on. His environment is also changed frequently by the entrance of other persons, each of whom produces a variety of stimuli for him to sense. A frequently changing environment, with many of the changes produced by the child himself, is an important facet of the foundation of language development.

In addition to its being stimulating, the child's environment must also be accepting. When parents and others respond to a child's gestures and vocalizations in a positive way and when they produce oral and body language for the child to see and hear, they help him learn that language has social utility. For many cerebral palsied children, the environment is neither adequately stimulating nor accepting. Because of their sensory-motor deficiencies, they are unable to produce the changes in their environment which create new experiences and, hence, new language-learning opportunities for them. Their restricted environments can produce only restricted language development. The limited attempts of some children to use symbolic behavior gives their parents few opportunities for positive responses to their child's language. Further, by being too accepting and by anticipating all his needs, some parents deny their child the reinforcements for his language learning which come from observing the effects of his language on his environment. Still other parents may have so much difficulty in accepting their cerebral palsied child that they virtually ignore him.

60 Do Schlanger's (159: 339-43) comments about the effect of environmental influences on verbal output of mentally retarded children support the recommendations of Westlake, and Rutherford (189), Mecham, Berko, and Berko (115), and Kastein (98: 4-19) regarding intensive early stimulation activities?

Time for Maturation and Learning

The third portion of our foundation for language development is time. The mere passage of time is not significant. Only as maturation and learning take place with the passage of time does language develop. Maturation and learning are interrelated. By *maturation* we mean the physical and physiological changes which occur in the nervous system and other parts of the body as the child grows older. By *learning* we mean those changes in the total function of the reaction mechanism which have come about through experience. To the extent that a child's physical and physiological level of development determines how he interacts with his environment, maturation must precede learning. Just as certain kinds of development precede other kinds of development in time, certain kinds of learning must precede other kinds of learning. In normal development, reflexes and reactions evolve as ascending levels of the central nervous system become dominant. The development of higher-level functions depends on the previous development of lower-level functions. This is also true of learned functions. Walking cannot be learned until the child has learned to stand. Vocalizing must precede babbling and babbling must precede the articulation of words. The development of cerebral palsied children often becomes arrested somewhere in the sequence and, if patterns above that level are learned at all, they are usually of poor quality.

SPEECH

Speech, one of the modalities for using language, is a series of movements whose end products are audible signals possessing communication value. Like all movements, the movements of speech are activated, monitored, and controlled by sensory and central processes. Speech production, then, is the function of a specialized reaction mechanism which operates basically as a closed-circuit servo-system. While it is often convenient to break speech production into sensory, central,

61   What is a servo-system and how does it operate in speech production?
      See Fairbanks (52: 133-39), Mysak (121: 144-49), McDonald (109).

and motor processes and to subdivide each of these processes, in reality the processes by which speech is produced are inextricably interrelated. Respiration, phonation, resonation, and articulation are effector processes by which audible signals are produced. A variety of sensations constitute receptor processes. Central functions include discrimination, coordination, and symbolization. The interrelationship of these processes is illustrated in Fig. 7. Any one of these processes might be disturbed in cerebral palsy, but usually one finds that several processes are involved when the cerebral palsied child has defective speech. The nature of the disturbance can best be understood by comparing abnormal with normal function.

It is to be remembered that in addition to their role in speech production the muscles which produce the movements of speech also perform some of the body's vegetative functions. The vegetative functions undergo marked modifications for the production of speech. In cerebral palsy, these modifications often do not occur and speech development is affected. To understand why some cerebral palsied children have difficulty in learning to talk, we should examine the *normal* characteristics of the processes by which speech is produced and then we should study these processes as they appear in cerebral palsy.

Respiration

Respiration is the process in which air flows into and out of the lungs, thus permitting the blood to absorb oxygen and to give off carbon dioxide and water. A simple physical principle accounts for the flow of air into and out of the lungs: gases flow from areas of high pressure to areas of low pressure. The walls of the thoracic cavity are movable, making possible variations in the volume of the cavity. Enlargement of the thoracic cavity through elevation of the rib cage and descent of the diaphragm increases the volume of the thoracic cavity

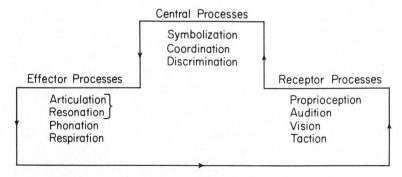

Figure 7. Reaction Mechanism for Production of Speech.

and consequently decreases the pressure of the gas contained therein to a level below that of atmospheric pressure. Air then flows into the lungs. Decrease in the size of the thoracic cavity through descent of the rib cage and ascent of the diaphragm reduces the volume and increases the pressure to a level greater than atmospheric pressure. The air now flows from the lungs. Descent of the diaphragm is accompanied by an increase in the abdominal circumference, hence both the thoracic and abdominal circumferences increase simultaneously in inhalation. Ascent of the diaphragm with lowering of the rib cage brings about a synchronous reduction in the circumferences of the thoracic and abdominal areas. In normal breathing, thoracic, diaphragmatic, and abdominal movements are coordinated. Normal rest breathing is rhythmic occurring at the rate of 16 to 20 cycles per minute. Inspiration and expiration are of approximately equal duration.

While breathing can be controlled voluntarily, respiration is basically a reflex function integrated at the brain-stem level. A respiratory center in the medulla activates the muscles of inspiration in response to a rise in the level of carbon dioxide concentration in the blood. Stretch receptors in lung tissues are activated by expansion of the lungs during inhalation and send impulses to the respiratory center which inhibit inhalation and allow exhalation to proceed. Receptors in the carotid and aortic bodies, sensitive to the chemical composition of the blood, also send impulses to the brain-stem respiratory center.

Exhalation provides the flow of air which is modified in the vocal tract to produce the audible speech signals. For the production of speech, vegetative breathing patterns undergo many changes. Instead of the rhythmic alternations of inhalation and exhalation, a quick inhalation precedes speech production and exhalations are prolonged. Superimposed on the larger movement of exhalation are patterns of movement which produce syllables, others which group the syllables into stress groups, or feet, and another pattern which combines the feet into breath-groups. Another movement of inhalation does not occur until the beginning of a new phrase. Since phrasing is related to the speaker's thought processes, it is likely that speech breathing is integrated at cortical levels but as an automatic, rather than voluntary, action.

In cerebral palsied children, several aberrations of breathing patterns are seen which seem to interfere with speech production. Too rapid a rate might make it difficult for the infant to indulge in the vocal play

---

62   For methods of evaluating breathing function see Darley (*35*), Westlake and Rutherford (*189*), Palmer (*128: 514*).

which is the antecedent of speech. In older children a rapid rate might prevent the prolongation of exhalation which is essential to speech production. Rates above 30 cycles per minute are often associated with

SPEECH BREATHING ANOMALIES AND ASSOCIATED SPEECH SYMPTOMS IN CEREBRAL PALSY

Breathing problem	*Associated speech symptoms*
Too rapid rate	Little vocalizing in infants
Difficulty in taking a deep inhalation	Often produces only one or two syllables on an exhalation Tension increases when longer vocalizations are tried
Difficulty in controlling a prolonged exhalatory movement	Difficulty in initiating vocalization Noticeable escape of air before initiation of vocalization Produces only a few syllables on an exhalation
Antagonistic diaphragmatic-abdominal and thoracic movements	Difficulty sustaining vocalization because of insufficient air if antagonism occurs on inhalation Interruption of vocalization if antagonism occurs during exhalation
Involuntary movements in respiratory musculature	Varied loudness of voice Interruptions of vocalization

poor speech production. Many cerebral palsied children are unable to take a deep breath voluntarily. As a rule, these children do not talk much and when they do attempt speech, they merely begin vocalizing with what air is available to them at the time. Asynchrony between the diaphragmatic-abdominal and the thoracic musculatures is commonly seen in cerebral palsied children. The thoracic musculature seems to be producing movements of inhalation, for example, while the abdominal musculature makes movements associated with exhalation. This condition is sometimes referred to as *reversed breathing*. At times the movement of exhalation might start with synchronous abdominal-thoracic movements but be interrupted by irregular movements in one or both of these areas. There are children who can take an adequately deep inhalation but cannot control the exhalation. They may exhale much of their air before beginning phonation or they may not be able to coordinate exhalation with their efforts to phonate.

63   After reviewing the reports of Blumberg (*13:* 48-53), Hardy (*76:* 309-19), Hull (*86:* 275-76), Mecham, Berko and Berko (*115*), and Westlake and Rutherford (*189*) concerning breathing problems in cerebral palsy, what more would you want to include in the table on this page?

Phonation

The larynx developed as a valve in the respiratory tract to protect the lungs from the entrance of undesirable material. Valving is achieved by a complex arrangement of cartilages and muscles which can bring together, at the midline, folds of tissues. Within the folds there are muscle fibers which are capable of regulating the tension of the folds. For rest breathing the vocal folds are abducted during both inhalation and exhalation. In speech breathing the vocal folds are abducted during inhalation and during the production of voiceless sounds. For the production of voiced sounds, the vocal folds are abducted. Most theories of sound production in the larynx suggest that the degree of tension in the vocal folds is related to both the intensity and the pitch of the voice.

Several types of laryngeal involvement are seen in children with cerebral palsy. An adductor spasm may hold the vocal folds together with such force that the child is unable to initiate phonation. The child will be observed to assume the articulatory positions for a sound such as a prolonged vowel or the first sound in *mama* but no sound is emitted. Failure to produce a phonation under these circumstances might be due either to an adductor spasm in the larynx or to an inability to initiate exhalation. To differentiate the cause, the examiner should have the child stripped to the waist and watch the thoracic area for signs of the initiation of a movement of exhalation. When the failure is due to a laryngeal block, it will be noted that the exhalatory movement is initiated but stopped. If the dysfunction is in the larynx the child can often produce the phonation if the position of his head is changed. Flexion, extension, or rotation of the head sometimes changes the laryngeal tension thus permitting phonation to begin. If the child is able to produce a tone when the head is being moved gently by the examiner, it is likely that the difficulty is an adductor spasm. Asking the child to vocalize at a different pitch level by giving him a pitch to imitate also is effective in some cases in breaking up an adductor laryngeal spasm. At times the adductor spasm is not present at the initiation of phonation but comes on during vocalization and thus abruptly interrupts phonation. In vegetative breathing lower levels of integration function to keep the larynx open and, during deglutition, they function to close the larynx; however, some cerebral palsied children must be fed with great care because of the danger of strangulation resulting from inefficient laryngeal valving during swallowing. Adductor spasms are most likely to occur when laryngeal function is integrated into the voluntary activity of speaking.

A second laryngeal problem found in cerebral palsied children is the abductor spasm which either prevents approximating the vocal folds for phonation or pulls the folds apart during phonation. When the folds are pulled apart during an abductor spasm, the voice becomes breathy and may have the quality of whispered speech. Uncontrollable variations in tension of the laryngeal muscles are also found in cerebral palsied children. These variations produce undesirable shifts in pitch intensity or voice quality.

> **64** After reviewing the work of Palmer (*131:* 40-41), Westlake (*188*), and Mecham, Berko and Berko (*115*) concerning laryngeal function in cerebral palsy, what changes would you make in the table on this page?

LARYNGEAL DYSFUNCTION AND ASSOCIATED SPEECH SYMPTOMS IN CEREBRAL PALSY

Laryngeal problem	*Associated speech symptoms*
Adductor spasm	If vocals folds are held tightly together, the child may have difficulty initiating phonation
	Phonation may be abruptly interrupted
Abductor spasm	Aspirate voice quality
Varying tension in laryngeal muscles	Voice may vary in pitch, intensity, or quality

Resonance and Articulation

Resonance and articulation are closely interrelated. Resonance is the physical process by which certain of the components of the complex tone produced at the larynx are damped or reinforced as they pass through the several cavities located in the vocal tract. Articulation is the physiological process by which the size, shape, and coupling of the oral-tract resonating cavities are modified and by which varying degrees of obstruction are placed in the way of the outgoing airstream, thus generating new patterns of sound. Since, through muscular action, the size, shape, and coupling of resonators are modifiable, aberrant patterns of neuromuscular function lead to resonance problems in cerebral palsied children. Generally, when the neuromuscular disturbance is severe enough to affect resonance, other processes involved in speech production will be disturbed and the resonance problem will be of secondary importance.

Articulation is achieved by coordinated movements of mandibular, labial, and lingual muscles. The vegetative use of these structures for chewing, sucking, and swallowing undergoes marked modification when the structures are employed for speech production. A major change is in the nature of the stimuli to which the sensory receptors of the lips, tongue, and jaw respond. At rest and during chewing, the lips are approximated, causing tactile stimuli to arise from broad surfaces of the lips. In sucking, a nipple or other object is intruded between the lips but still, throughout its length, each lip is in contact either with the other lip or with the intruding object. At rest, during sucking, and during chewing, the lips are approximated or are in contact with a nipple for long periods, thus giving rise to continuous tactile stimulation. In speaking, the lips are separated for varying periods of time and by varying degrees, thus a rapidly changing pattern of stimulation arises from the lips during speaking periods. In crying the lips are separated, hence, for long periods little tactile stimulation arises from the lips.

At rest the tongue, over much of its surface, is in contact with other portions of the oral cavity. During chewing and drinking the tongue is also stimulated over much of its superior surface because the liquids and food particles tend to be distributed widely over the lingual area. Not only do these patterns of stimulation cover a large lingual surface, but they change slowly. For speaking, the tongue loses its broad surface contacts with stimulating agents and is very selectively stimulated, as when the tip of the tongue touches the teeth or the back of the tongue makes contact with the palate. Again, instead of broad stimulation of long duration and slow change, in speech the stimuli are of short duration and shift rapidly from place to place.

In chewing, the muscles of mastication must produce sufficient force to break up the food and must operate together in such a way as to produce the grinding pattern characteristic of mastication. The rotary-like movements of chewing are not so observable in the mandibular activity associated with talking, and there is no need for as much strength of contraction. The difference in strength and pattern of movement would, of course, give rise to different patterns of sensation from the muscles of mastication.

Normal speech is characterized by simultaneous movements of different parts of the articulatory mechanism or, as in the case of the tongue, within the same mechanism. Temporal overlapping is seen in the movements of the lips and tongue when saying "u*p d*ad" and overlapping movements occur in different parts of the tongue when saying *sk* in "ask." Temporal overlapping of movements of various portions of the articulatory mechanism is not so dominant a characteristic of chewing, sucking, and swallowing activities. The character of overlapping movements becomes increasingly complex as the child progresses from producing simple consonant-vowel combinations in his vocal play to the production of abutting consonants in the jargon and two-word-sentence stages of speech development.

65 What are simple, compound, and abutting consonants and by what kind of articulatory movements are they produced? See McDonald (*109*) and Stetson (*171*).

Poor mandibular, labial, and lingual coordination is often seen in cerebral palsied children. Some children, even in the presence of an adequate airway for respiration, seem to have difficulty maintaining the mandible sufficiently elevated to keep their mouths closed. Others have difficulty controlling the range of mandibular movement. In normal connected speech the mandible is rarely lowered as much as 20 millimeters from its rest position; however, it moves rapidly and frequently within this range to assume positions appropriate for the production of different speech sounds. In cerebral palsied children, one frequently sees a hyperdepression of the mandible which is sometimes so extreme as to cause the condyle of the mandible to slip out of the temporomandibular fossa. This condition is known as a *mandibular facet slip*. Overdepression of the mandible interferes with speech production by pulling

66 Review the anatomy and physiology relating to normal mandibular function, Kaplan (*96*), and determine the various mechanisms by which the mandibular condyle slips from the glenoid fossa in some cerebral palsied patients. See Palmer (*130*: 44-48).

the tongue into a position which makes lingual-dental and lingual-palatal contacts difficult or impossible and changes the resonating cavity relationships, thus causing speech sounds to have unintelligible and unpleasant characteristics.

Labial control is often affected in cerebral palsied children. Many children are unable to keep the lips approximated at rest and they may have difficulty with protruding and retracting the lips. Drooling is common in these children and feeding is difficult. They cannot make a seal around a nipple or straw for sucking, they have difficulty in closing the lips for swallowing when drinking from a glass, and they have difficulty in keeping the lips approximated while chewing, hence, large amounts of food and liquid escape from the mouth. Sounds requiring lip approximation or labiodental contacts are usually misarticulated by children who have poor labial coordination.

Normally the tongue can assume many positions and shapes. For speech production, movements of protrusion, elevation of the tongue tip, retroflexion of the tongue tip, and elevation of the back of the tongue are important. These movements must be precisely coordinated with movements of the mandible and of the lips, and movements of different parts of the tongue must be coordinated with each other. Further, for normal articulation it is important to be able to move the tongue independently of the lips and mandible.

While not important for speech production, lateral movements of the tip of the tongue are employed in eating to manipulate the bolus of food between the teeth and to remove food from the buccal sulcus. Some cerebral palsied children are seen who seem to be incapable of any movement of the tongue on a voluntary level and who have only minimal reflex tongue activity. On examination, the tongue appears to be a large, inert mass of tissue. More common, however, is their inability to elevate or retroflex the tongue tip. Since approximately 85 per cent of the consonants used in continuous speech require some degree of elevation or retroflexion of the tongue tip, inability to elevate the tongue has a markedly detrimental effect on speech production. Children are also seen who can produce diadochokinetic movements of the tongue tip but are unable to perform the more complicated overlapping movements which are essential for normal speech production. When athetoid movements are present in the tongue, speech sounds are often so distorted that they are unrecognizable.

Normally there is a balance between the masticatory, labial, and lingual muscles which operates to help mold the bony configuration of the oral area. In cerebral palsied children, this balance is disturbed and marked oral anomalies are frequently seen. Marked deformities of the upper dental arch and palate occur in children who from infancy sit with the mouth open and lips separated, thus providing no counterforce to the strong protrusive movements of the tongue. By the time they have attained their permanent dentition, some of these children are unable to approximate the lips because of the extreme anterior growth of the upper dental arch. Such a malocclusion is obviously detrimental to speaking, feeding, and cosmetics.

67   After reviewing the work of Palmer (128: 514), Westlake and Rutherford
      (189), Mecham, Berko, and Berko (115), Mysak (124: 252-60), and Hardy,
      (76: 309-19), what additions would you make to the chart on page 95?

ASSESSING LANGUAGE DEVELOPMENT

Frequently in treatment centers the speech and hearing therapist will encounter children who have very limited means of communication. Before attempting to help these children develop communication skills,

COMMON PROBLEMS IN LINGUAL, MANDIBULAR, AND LABIAL CONTROL AND THEIR ASSOCIATED VEGETATIVE AND ARTICULATORY DIFFICULTIES

Mandible	Weakness in elevators	Mouth usually open, drooling common, chewing pattern poor, articulation often defective
	Hyperactive depressors	Hyperextension of mandible during eating and speaking, when extreme, causes mandibular facet slip
Lips	Weakness	Difficulty in protruding or retracting lips or in maintaining bilabial approximation, poor sucking pattern, drools
	Involuntary motion	Patterns of lip movements not predictable, sucking pattern not normal
Tongue	Immobile with practically no ability to perform voluntary movements	Sucking, swallowing, and chewing difficult, drooling common, speech consists primarily of a few vowels.
	Performs only gross movements with no voluntary elevation of tongue tip	Sucking, swallowing, and chewing difficult but developing, speech consists primarily of vowel sounds, but some consonantal approximations are present
	Voluntary movement possible but slow and poorly coordinated	Sucking, swallowing, and chewing patterns present but not normal, speech includes consonants, but they are often misarticulated
	Involuntary movements	Sucking, swallowing, and articulation are unpredictable
	Movements not independent of labial and mandibular movements	Sucking, swallowing, and chewing patterns usually developed but not normal, articulatory movements slow and nonspecific

it is essential for the therapist to determine what language concepts the child has developed. Also before beginning therapy, it is essential to know to what extent the child can follow simple instructions and how well he hears and discriminates auditory stimuli. For this purpose, the following set of tasks which require only that the child indicate yes or no or that he look in the correct direction has been arranged. If the child can manipulate his head best in a horizontal plane, the objects and pictures may be arranged on a table so that the examiner can tell at which one the child is looking. If the child is to respond by pointing, it is essential to consider where the pictures and objects can best be placed in order for him to see them. If the child can control the head and eyes best in a vertical plane, the objects and pictures may be hung on a board where the child can most easily see it. A large cooky sheet and magnetic hangers provide a flexible arrangement for displaying the materials. The hangers can be positioned to take advantage of the child's best controlled patterns of movement; however, they must be kept sufficiently separated to allow the therapist to determine at which object or picture the child is looking or pointing. *The following items do not constitute a scale.* By themselves, they do not indicate the child's potential for learning language or developing speech. Their basic use is to help determine at what language level the therapist might communicate with the child.

Following Simple Instructions

1. *Single instruction*
    Look at the light.
    Open your mouth.
    Show me your foot.
    Where's Momma (or Daddy)?
    Look at (name favorite toy which has been placed to one side).
2. *Ability to follow two instructions*
    Look at the door, then show me your shoe.
    Show me your hand, then look at my foot.
    Move your foot (or hand) and then shake your head.

The average two year old can carry out one instruction and the average three year old can carry out two instructions of the type given above.

Concepts

1. *Recognition of common objects*
    Arrange the following common objects before the child and ask him to look at each one: spoon, cup, knife, doll, comb, watch, pencil.

The average two year old will be able to recognize three objects and the average three year old can recognize five objects.

2. *Recognition of body parts*
   Hold a large doll or a drawing of a doll where the child can see it and ask him to look at the doll's hair, then the doll's head and the doll's feet.

The average two and a half year old can identify these three parts.

3. *Recognition of familiar objects by use*
   Arrange appropriately before the child a toy stove, a toy chair, a toy bed and a toy car, and then ask the child to:
   Look at what we ride in.
   Look at the one we sleep in.
   Look at the one we sit in.
   Look at the one we cook on.

The average two and a half year old recognizes three of these objects by use.

4. *Recognition of colors*
   a. *Matching*
      Place a red square, a blue square, a green square, and a yellow square where the child can see them. Then, one at a time, show him matching squares and ask him to look at the one which is the same.

The average three-year-old child matches three colors.

   b. *Recognition of color by name*
      Place the colored squares as in (a) and, one at a time, ask the child to look at the red square, the blue square, the green square, and the yellow square.

The average four year old recognizes these colors by name.

5. *Common information*
   Determine how the child indicates *yes* and *no,* then ask the following questions:
   a. Is your name John Jones? Is your name Bill Smith? Is your name (then give the child's name)?

For a girl, use girl's names. The average two year old recognizes his name. After four years, a child will smile or in some other way indicate that he thinks it is funny when names of the wrong sex are used.

   b. Are you a boy (or a girl)?

    c. Are you one year old? Are you four years old? Are you two
years old? Are you three years old?

The average three-year-old child responds correctly to questions
about his sex and his age. Beginning at about six years of age, children
indicate that they think there is something absurd about questions as:
Are you twenty-one years of age? Are you married?

    d. Is it nighttime?
    e. Did you have candy for breakfast?

The average four-year-old child can answer these questions.

  6. *Understanding of prepositions*
      Assemble four small box-and-ball sets as follows: Attach a ball
to the inside of a box which has no top so that the child can see
the ball in the box; attach a ball to the top of a box; attach a ball
to the side of a box; attach a ball to the bottom of a box. Place
the four sets where the child can see them and say:
      Look at the ball that is in the box.
      Look at the ball that is on the box.
      Look at the ball that is under the box.
      Look at the ball that is beside the box.

The average three-year-old child will know one or two of these
prepositions and the average four year old will understand three or
four.

  7. *Size and quantity*
    a. Place two boxes, one large and one small, where the child can
see them and say, "Look at the big box." Rearrange the boxes
and ask the child to look at the little box. Give several trials
changing the position of the boxes each time and ask the child
to look at either the big or the little box.

The average three and a half year old will look at the correct box
most of the time.

    b. In a matter-of-fact tone of voice, say to the child:
      You have more hands than feet, haven't you?
      Do you have more legs than a dog?
      You have as much candy as a candy store, haven't you?
      Does a bicycle have as many wheels as a car?

The average child between four and five years of age would respond
correctly to the statements about quantity.

There are many other concepts which a therapist might ask for, but these give the therapist some basis for determining the level and in what areas communication might be established with the child. The ages cited are rough approximations in some instances. With these

> 68   For additional suggestions concerning the evaluation of cerebral palsied children see Allen and Jefferson (2), Mecham, Berko, and Berko (115), Wood (191), Westlake and Rutherford (189), and Taylor (176).

qualifications made clear to the other members of the rehabilitation group, the therapist might cautiously speak of a child's ability to follow simple instructions as being poorer than that of the two year old, like that of a two year old, or like that of a three year old. Again observing the necessary qualifications, the therapist might, on the basis of these tasks, compare the child's language concepts to those of children two, three, or four years of age. These observations when added to the observations of other members of the staff will provide an estimate of the child's present level of functioning.

ORAL COMMUNICATION DEVELOPMENT

Information about the oral communication abilities of the child will be useful in many ways. When added to other information about the child, information about his communication abilities will contribute to an over-all assessment of his developmental level. Knowledge about his communication abilities will be helpful to teachers, therapists, and others who must communicate with the child; an assessment of his development of oral communication skills will give the speech therapist some indication of what skills need attention. It should be remembered that in working with young cerebral palsied children, it is more important to identify functions which the child has already learned and those with which he needs helps than to classify a child according to an index such as a language age. In order to determine if oral communication skills are being learned at a normal rate, the therapist should be familiar with normal developmental sequences. For assessing the oral speech development of cerebral palsied children, the developmental period may be roughly divided into the following six stages. These stages overlap to some extent and the child may be developing skills in more than one stage at the same time. However, mastery of the stages occurs approximately in the indicated order. *This outline does not constitute a speech-development scale.* The ages given are to be regarded as approximations rather than as norms. They provide only a rough indication of the age at which the average child begins the skill indicated.

1. *Undifferentiated vocalizations*

   The first vocalizations of the infant consist of crying and other reflexive sounds. During the first two weeks of life, most of the infant's vocalizations occur during hunger, pain, or other discomfort. The vocalizations tend to be very similar, varying only in loudness and duration. The nature of the child's discomfort cannot be determined from the type of vocalization.

2. *Differentiated vocalizations*

   Around the end of the first month the infant vocalizes in different ways to express hunger, pain, and various types of discomfort such as uncomfortable positions or restrictive clothing.

3. *Babbling and vocal play*

   Where crying is associated with feelings of discomfort, babbling and vocal play are associated with feelings of relief and contentment. The infant seems to derive pleasure from babbling and accompanies it with many other movements of his body. At about two months the infant plays with the vocalization of a single vowel by varying its pitch and loudness. He soon adds many vowels to his repertoire. By four months of age, the infant produces many consonant-vowel combinations. At first he makes only one consonant-vowel at a time, but by six months of age he can produce several syllables on an exhalation. During his first year the normal child will have practiced all the sounds of his language plus many other sounds. Sometime between the seventh and ninth months the average child begins practicing inflections. His vocalizations will follow patterns of questioning, exclaiming, commanding, and many others, some of which are not identifiable.

4. *Socialized vocalization*

   At about the fifth month, the normal infant begins to vocalize to attract attention. He begins to associate his primitive vocalizations with demands for something he wants and with rejection of things he does not want. He is learning that through vocalizing he can express himself and modify the behavior of others. The average nine-month-old child can imitate the vocalizations produced by his mother or father.

5. *Symbolic use of words*

   Eager parents often date the child's first word from the accidental doubling of the syllable *ma* to say *"mama"* or the syllable *da* to say *"dada."* Not until the child uses his vocalization to symbolize his mother or father can the vocalization be truly called a word. At about one year of age, the average child begins learning the names of objects. His early vocabulary will consist predominantly of nouns; however, some action words are acquired beginning shortly after one year. At about two years of age the child begins using pronouns especially *I, me,* and *you.* His vocabulary grows from approximately three words from one year to twenty words at a year and a half and more than two-hundred words by two years of age. During the third year the child learns to make plural nouns, to form the past tense of verbs, and to use modifiers and prepositions.

6. *Sentences*

The child's first sentences consist of one word and depend largely on intonation for their meaning. Thus the child may say "up" to indicate that he wants someone to pick him up or he may say "milk" to indicate that he is hungry and wants someone to give him his lunch. Between eighteen months and two years, the normal child begins combining a noun and a verb to make a two-word sentence. At two and a half he begins adding another word to his simple sentence. Between three and four years of age, the child learns to use a conjunction to combine two simple sentences into a compound sentence and at about the same time he begins making complex sentences.

When the child has not yet developed symbolic use of words, it is necessary through careful interviewing of the parents or someone else who is familiar with the child to establish the type of vocalizations which the child employs. It is not unusual to find cerebral palsied children and even adolescents who are incapable of producing differentiated vocalizations and who have never enjoyed vocal play.

69   For an interesting popular account of speech development see Van Riper *(180)*. Also see Irwin and Chen *(91:* 109-21), Templin *(177),* and Gesell *(63).*

By creating situations in which the child is encouraged to talk, the therapist can get much useful information about the level of the child's speech and language development through observing the forms of the sentences he uses. If the child's speech development is below what would be expected of a child his age, the therapist should not assume that his language development is also limited. The language abilities of inarticulate cerebral palsied children should be assessed through procedures which do not require a verbal response from them.

We recently evaluated a five-year-old child who, with a great deal of effort, could sometimes produce a short phonation. Her severe upper-extremity involvement precluded any use of her hands for accurate pointing. The therapists and teachers who had been working with her for two months felt that she was severely mentally retarded and unresponsive to verbal stimulation. Experimentation demonstrated that she could move her head and eyes in a horizontal plane. By asking her to look at one of two objects held where she could see them by turning her head, it was possible to demonstrate that she knew the prepositions in, on, and beside; could identify objects by use, knew her age, and had other common information.

Testing Hearing for Above-Threshold Sounds

The comprehensive work-up which every cerebral palsied child must have should include audiologic studies. Sometimes these are not available and often even when they can be arranged, there is considerable delay before the studies are made. Before beginning to treat the child, however, the speech therapist needs to know how he responds to familiar sounds. With the child who is not developing articulate speech it is especially important to determine if he responds to noises and to speech at conversational levels. The following observations will provide some clues to the child's response to sound.

Gross Responses

Infants respond to a loud, sudden noise with a startle reaction consisting of a jerking movement of some parts of the body. This reaction may be elicited in many older cerebral palsied children in response to a loud noise. Beginning at about four months the normal child will turn his head on hearing a familiar sound such as his mother's voice or the clinking of his bottle. To check the ability of the young cerebral palsied child to hear his mother's voice, the therapist might hold the child in his arms with his back to the mother so that the therapist can see the child's face, but the child cannot see his mother. When the mother calls the child's name in a conversational level voice, the therapist should watch the child's head and eyes for signs that the child is trying to find his mother.

The average six-month-old child is learning to localize sound and will look in the direction from which a noise came. To test this ability in the cerebral palsied child, the therapist might engage the child in some activity, such as looking at pictures or playing with "silly putty," while an assistant rings a bell in different parts of the room, being careful not to provide the child with visual clues as to her whereabouts. The ability of the child to identify certain noisemakers can be checked by placing where a child can see them, a bell, whistle, horn, rattle, squeaky mouse, and a gun. Using duplicates of these objects, demonstrate for the child the noise made by each. From behind a screen which obscures your actions from the child, produce a noise with one of the duplicate noisemakers and ask the child to look at or point to the toy which makes a noise of that type. In this way the therapist should present all of the noises to the child. With some children it will be possible to have no more than two or three toys displayed at a time.

Discrimination of Speech Sounds

To determine how well the child can differentiate vowel sounds, place before him pictures of a ball, bowl, bell, bull, and tell him the name of each picture if he does not know it. With your face obscured from his view ask him to point to or look at the picture you name. Additional combinations to be tried are pen, pin, pan; bat, boot, boat, beet; ship, sheep.

The following combinations may be used in the same way to determine the child's ability to differentiate consonants: boat, goat; ball, doll; block, clock; tie, pie; bear, pear.

Steps in Preliminary Language and Speech Evaluation

While the techniques just described produce some useful information about the cerebral palsied child's intellectual status and about his auditory functioning, they do not take the place of an adequate psychological or an adequate audiological evaluation. As indicators of intelligence or audiological status, we might put them in the category of "what to do until the audiologist and psychologist come." These procedures are intended primarily, however, to aid the speech therapist make the following determinations which are essential to planning a program of speech training.

1. Determine the status of the child's language and speech development.
   a. What language does the child understand?
      If a child two years of age or older appears, after repeated observations, to be unresponsive to spoken language, the possibility of aphasia, auditory impairment, and mental retardation should be investigated. If the child seems to understand language but not as well as other children of his age, the possibility of lack of opportunities to gain experiences should also be explored.
   b. What speech does the child use?
      If the child understands language but has not developed the

expected level of speech skills, it is necessary to differentiate between an expressive language difficulty (expressive aphasia) and a motor problem (dysarthria).

2. Determine how the reaction mechanism for speech production functions.

   a. Receptor
      1) What environmental sounds, including speech, does the child hear? Between which does he discriminate?
      2) Does the child respond to tactile stimuli in and around the oral cavity?
   b. Effector
      1) Is respiratory control adequately developed for speech production?
      2) Does uncontrolled laryngeal activity interfere with speech production?
      3) Are labial, lingual, and mandibular movements adequately developed and controlled for articulating?
   c. Central
      1) Are the interactions of respiration, phonation, and articulation adequately coordinated for the production of speech?

It is to be remembered that diagnosis of the child's problem will not be refined and established by the efforts of one member of the rehabilitation group, but by staff review of medical, psychological, audiological, and other special studies, plus an evaluation of the child's response to treatment.

>   70   How does this outline for making a preliminary language and speech evaluation relate to the foundations of language development and to the reaction mechanism for speech production described earlier in this chapter?

What are the speech and language problems of the cerebral palsied children described in Chapter I? Using the information given for Charles Pounka, Clayton Penths, Charleen Pimskon, Catherine Pombst, Carl Pednok, and Clifford Puzin, can you describe the status of their language and speech development? Which, if any, of them seem to have symptoms of aphasia? Why, at four years of age, was Clifford often unable to make a sound even though he obviously was trying? Analyze the receptor and effector function of each child as fully as you can from their case descriptions.   ᒋᒋᒋ

TO THE QUESTION, "WHEN SHOULD SPEECH AND LANGUAGE TRAINING for a cerebral palsied child begin?," our answer is simple and direct, "As soon as it is suspected that the child might be cerebral palsied!" This response is based on the following assumptions about the early origin of language and speech problems of many severely involved cerebral palsied children:

1. Language development is basic to speech development.
2. Experience is essential for language development.
3. The sensory-motor dysfunction of the cerebral palsied child interferes with gaining experience through interactions with his environment.
4. Deprivation of experience adversely affects both the cerebral palsied child's ability to develop concepts about which he can talk and his awareness of the social utility of language and speech.

language and speech
problems: treatment

5. Modification of vegetative breathing to permit controlled, prolonged exhalations is essential for speech development.
6. Control of laryngeal valving is necessary for speech development.
7. Ability to produce independent yet temporally overlapping movements of the lips, tongue, mandible, and velum is fundamental to the development of speech.
8. The reaction mechanism by which speech is produced functions as a unitary system. The ability to coordinate the processes of respiration, phonation, and articulation is basic to speech development.
9. Impaired tactile-kinesthetic function within the speech-producing mechanism may interfere with the development of motor skills.
10. Failure to develop higher-level motor integrations with resultant dominance of lower-level motor integrations interferes with speech development.
11. Delay in developing speech sometimes interferes with the development of language.
12. Failure to develop language and speech might be the result of mental retardation, aphasia, or severe auditory impairment in the cerebral palsied child.
13. Potential causes of language and speech problems may exist in varying degrees and in various combinations.
14. Having a handicapped child gives rise to many natural parental reactions some of which are unwholesome. Unless these reactions

are understood and properly managed they may interfere with the child's development.

These assumptions lead to the recommendation that if a cerebral palsied child is not indulging in vocal play and is not responsive to spoken language by the time he is about eighteen months old he should be started on a program of language-stimulation and speech-development activities. If the child is a severe athetoid, a rigidity, or a spastic quadriplegic, the therapist should have frequent conferences with the parents to guide them in carrying out a program of language stimulation and speech training. While paraplegics and hemiplegics are less likely to have language and speech problems, all young cerebral palsied children should be observed frequently by the speech therapist, and a training program should be initiated for any infant or child whose language and speech development are not progressing satisfactorily.

Unfortunately, however, the speech therapist usually does not get to see the cerebral palsied child or his parents until the child is three or four years of age. For the child with severe motor involvement this is two or three years too late.

Early and continuing stimulation to counteract the sensory deprivation resulting from his motor dysfunction is an important part of the language- and speech-training program for cerebral palsied children. Many of the training procedures can be incorporated into the routines of feeding, dressing, toileting, bathing, and playing with the child. Parents need the guidance of a speech therapist to plan and carry out these procedures effectively. It is the responsibility of the speech therapist to convince physicians and other members of the rehabilitation group of the importance and feasibility of early language stimulation and speech training for cerebral palsied children.

71　What are the psychological problems which a therapist should be aware of in "making mother a clinician"? See Bice (11), McDonald (108), Wortis (192: 8-9), Lillywhite (106: 61-66).

While the fourteen assumptions listed at the beginning of this chapter seem to be related primarily to the speech and language problems of young, severely involved cerebral palsied children, they apply to older children also. It is to be remembered that older children were once younger and that their speech and language problems are reflections of concepts which they failed to learn or sensory-motor skills which they failed to develop at earlier stages of maturation and learning. With the older cerebral palsied child it is often necessary to begin therapy at a very primitive level such as breaking up or weakening infantile oral-reflex patterns which interfere with the development of articulatory movements. One of the weaknesses of many speech therapy programs for older cerebral palsied patients is that the techniques are directed toward developing higher-order speech skills before lower-level functions have been adequately developed.

It would seem obvious that therapy should be directed to the problems identified by systematic diagnosis and appraisal. Yet, too often, therapists are inclined to begin treating the older cerebral palsied child without first determining what parts of the speech-production process need attention and in what order. As a result, many hours are spent futilely working on articulation skills with a cerebral palsied child who can't consistently produce a controlled exhalation. The result is no better than that achieved by a mechanic who adjusts the car-buretor in an effort to improve the operation of an automobile when the fuel pump is defective. Both the therapist and the mechanic get paid, of course, but the mechanic will soon get a complaint. Who complains about the therapist? Hopefully, the therapist will become his own effective critic.

It would be impossible to tell you how to treat a cerebral palsied child. As the brief descriptions of the six children introduced in Chapter I demonstrate, the problems of individual cerebral palsied children vary markedly, hence, therapy plans must be devised individually. In previous chapters we have tried to help you recognize and understand the problems of cerebral palsied children. Our objective in this chapter is to provide a source of information and rationale which will guide the therapist in working on the problems suggested by our fourteen assumptions. The techniques described are meant to be illustrative. Many more should be added to your repertoire through wide reading and the exercise of your own creativity. Remember, though, that every technique you use should be related to your diagnosis, have a rationale, and be based on sound principles of motor learning.

DEVELOPING LANGUAGE: PROBLEMS AND ILLUSTRATIVE TECHNIQUES

The earlier a systematic program of language stimulation is provided for the cerebral palsied child the more effective it is likely to be. Most of the suggested activities would be carried out by the parents, but they should be closely supervised by the therapist who, in addition to guiding the mother's efforts, would also be alert for signs of aphasia, hearing loss, mental retardation, or any other factor which might interfere with language development. Aphasic children or children with severe hearing losses should have appropriate training programs.

Heighten the Child's Awareness of Receptor Function and Relate Sensations to the Source of Stimulation

The infant's mouth is an important source of sensations and experience during the first year. Unfortunately many mothers are so concerned about their cerebral palsied child that feeding is an unpleasant ordeal. With guidance the mother can be taught to employ techniques during feeding which will heighten the child's awareness of the stimuli aroused and help him identify these sensations with his environment. For example, the mother should withdraw the nipple frequently and hold the bottle and nipple where the child can see it. After the child has seen the nipple, instead of pushing it quickly into the child's mouth, she should tease him, holding it before him and then touching it against his lips, repeating this several times. Feeding in front of a mirror will help the child see the relationship between the sensations in his mouth and the nipple. When soft foods are added to the child's diet, the mother should follow the same procedures with the spoon and baby-food jars. Parents should be taught to capitalize on the young child's tendency to "put everything into his mouth" by helping him mouth blocks, rattles, and so on.

Early in infancy the hands of the normal child become a source of pleasant sensory experiences. He sucks his fingers and fist, watches his hand as he holds it before him and moves it about, and later uses his hands to contact, grasp, and manipulate objects. In playing with the cerebral palsied child, a mother can help him use his hands in these ways. She might brush the child's fist against his face as she moves it into contact with his mouth. Bringing the child's hands together in his line of vision and patting and rubbing them together as in playing pat-a-cake will give rise to visual, tactile, and kinesthetic sensations.

72 Westlake (*188*) and Westlake and Rutherford (*189*) recommend heightening the child's awareness of stimuli, while Mysak (*123*: 221-30) recommends desensitizing the child. How do you reconcile these two recommendations?

Awareness of the source of auditory sensations should be stimulated by activities such as shaking a rattle in the child's line of vision and holding him so that he can see his bottle as it is set, with an audible noise, on a table or stand.

Visual stimulation is involved in many of the techniques just described. Hanging a mirror over the child's bed will enable him to see his movements. Placing a large tin pan in his bed and then manipulating his hand or foot to bump the pan will simultaneously give rise to visual, tactile, kinesthetic, and auditory stimuli.

Provide Many Opportunties for Interaction with the Environment

The environment of the normal child expands rapidly. When he learns to roll over, he can change his tactile environment. With each gain in motor control he increases his opportunities for interacting with his environment. The mobility he achieves through crawling and later through walking give him countless opportunities to be aroused by a variety of environmental stimuli. The cerebral palsied child is apt to remain in the supine position; so, his parents should be advised to help him roll over periodically so that he can lie on his side or stomach. The position of his head, arms, and legs should be varied from time to time. Instead of lying in the crib all the time, he should be placed on the floor or on a couch. And all of these things should not be done silently. The mother should verbalize what she is doing—and in the language of love. Before he is able to sit by himself, he should be held with his head in an upright position so that he can look around. Later, special seating should be arranged, if necessary, to provide needed support for sitting.

Especial attention should be given to providing the child with opportunities to differentiate between stimuli. Holding a rattle and a bell before the child and sounding them alternately will help him hear the differences between them. Later the child can be taught through frequent opportunities for observation, the differences between the sound of the sweeper and the TV set, the telephone and the dog barking, etc. The mother should help the child learn to localize sound by speaking to him from different parts of the room while he is lying in his crib. When he is old enough the infant should have an opportunity to experience different temperatures through frequent trips to other parts of the house or outdoors. Later, warm objects and cold objects might be placed in his hands and against his lips. Always these should be accompanied by a running commentary of pleasant sound from the parent.

Stimulate and Encourage Vocalization

Vocalization is important to language development because it is a primitive form of one of the child's earliest methods of using language. Speech, which develops from vocalizations, provides the child with an important tool for self-expression. Techniques for stimulating vocalization will be described in the section dealing with speech development.

Develop an Awareness of the Social Utility of Language

Once a child realizes that the noises or gestures he makes bring about desired responses from people in his environment, he is likely to expand his repertoire of signals. Through repeated effective use the symbolic value of the signals increases. Complete anticipation of the child's needs precludes his need for signaling. Parents of the cerebral palsied child should be taught to wait until the child informs them that he is hungry before feeding him or that he is wet before diapering him. They should be taught to listen for and to respond appropriately to differentiations in his vocalization. Parents should be taught that if they chatter constantly to their cerebral palsied child, he will respond to their speech as mere noise and attach only the grossest meaning to it. Speech should be used selectively so that the child has opportunities to associate the noises with events in his environment.

Develop Concepts

The first language concepts of the child are concrete and consist initially of names attached to people or things in his environment. His understanding of language precedes his ability to express it.

The cerebral palsied child's parents should help him learn the names of familiar objects. As they turn the light on in his darkened room, they should say "light" as they hold him facing the light fixture. They should darken the room and repeat this procedure. This should be done until the child will look at the light source when the word *light* is spoken to him. When the mother gives the baby his bottle she should hold it before him and clearly say "milk." Instead of letting him suck until he has had his fill, she should withdraw the nipple and again, holding the bottle where the child can see it, say "milk." It is important that these words be spoken as isolated words and that there be brief periods of silence preceding and following them. Later, a large photographic portrait of the mother should be obtained and the mother would

---

73   For techniques to be used with older children see Barry (7), Kastein (98: 4-19), McGinnis (110), and Plotkin (147: 16-20).

---

show this to the child and say "mama." This should be done until the child will look at the portrait or his mother when someone asks, "Where's mama?" A picture of the father can be used in the same way and later pictures of siblings. When feeding the child with a spoon, his mother should frequently hold the spoon where he can see it and say "spoon"—and say it fondly. Beginning at about one year of age, the child should be told the names of common objects: bed, chair, table, stove, and so forth. Even before he is ready to say these words, he should learn to respond to such questions as "where is the chair?" by looking at it. When the child is approximately two years of age, his mother should frequently sit before a large mirror and, when pointing to his eye, say "eye." She should then hold his hand and point a finger toward his eye while again saying, "eye." In this way the child would be taught to point to the parts of his body as they are being named. Later he should be shown these parts on a doll and on his mother. A later step would be to ask him to point to the doll's eye, his eye, or mama's eye. Sometime between two and three years of age, a photograph of the child can be used to help him learn his name and the pronoun *me*. Good snapshots taken of the child while eating, drinking, sleeping, sitting, and playing may be used to teach the child action words.

74   "Parallel talking"—an effective stimulant of language development—is a method used by the mother to attempt to verbalize the thoughts of the child. See Van Riper (181) and Levinson (105: 253-57).

IMPROVING BREATHING PATTERNS: PROBLEMS AND ILLUSTRATIVE TECHNIQUES

Speech therapists have often been inclined to attempt to teach speech breathing to cerebral palsied children by starting with blowing and phonation. While these techniques may have a small place in the treatment of cerebral palsied children, they are often inappropriate until more basic skills are learned. Too often, also, work on breathing patterns is not started until the child is of nursery-school age or older. Actually, if possible, attention should be given to the development of adequate speech-breathing patterns before the child is a year old. The following techniques will prove helpful in developing or improving breathing patterns for speech. They require the close cooperation of the physical therapist, speech therapist, and parent.

Break Up Persistent Tonic Reflex Patterns

Abnormal distribution of muscle tone in the abdominal, thoracic, and neck muscles is often found in children who have inadequate speech-breathing patterns. When strong tonic reflexes persist they should be weakened or broken up through systematic use of such techniques as reflex inhibition or sensory facilitation.

> 75   Review reflex inhibition and facilitation as described by Mysak (122),
>   Crickmay (29), and Marland (144: 111-19). Why would it be advisable
>   for the physical therapist and the speech therapist to work closely to-
>   gether when employing these procedures?

Facilitate Developmental Sequences Which Lead to Good Sitting Posture

The sitting posture of many cerebral palsied children makes the development of an adequate speech-breathing pattern difficult. They seem to collapse because much of the weight of the trunk and head bears down on the abdominal area, thus interfering with function of the diaphragm and abdominal musculature. The back is rounded and the head is flexed so that the chin rests on the chest. In this position elevation of the rib cage for inhalation is difficult. Neuromotor organization for sitting develops in a cephalocaudal direction. Gaining control of muscles of the head and neck area must be achieved before the head can be held erect; this also permits compensations for changes in bodily posture. Treatment directed toward taking a child through the developmental sequences leading to unsupported sitting with good posture is basic to a program for developing speech breathing.

Maintaining Proper Postural Relationships between Abdomen, Trunk, Neck, and Head

When the development of unsupported sitting with good posture is delayed, it is quite likely that children will be held in someone's lap or allowed to sit supported by pillows, belts, or other devices. Marked flexion of the head, chest, and abdominal areas is characteristic of such sitting. Prolonged sitting in this position leads to poor breathing habits. Seating in a properly fitted and adjusted rélaxation chair will help the child maintain a more satisfactory postural relationship between the head, neck, trunk, and abdominal areas. When an extensor thrust occurs during vocalizing, flexion at the hips by decreasing the angle at which the seat of the relaxation chair is attached to the back often reduces the strength of the extensor pattern. The normal child is capable of unsupported sitting by about seven months of age. If a cerebral palsied child cannot sit unsupported with good posture by the time he is twelve months of age, consideration should be given to the use of adequate seating equipment as well as to a program of developmental training. Initially the back of the chair should be tilted back from the 90-degree angle until the child can sit without slumping forward. As he gains head, neck, and trunk control through physical therapy, the angle of the back of the chair should be gradually changed until the child can sit in an upright position. In physical therapy, attention must be given to the flexors of the neck and shoulders as well as to the extensor muscles. While the extensors are used to maintain an upright position of the head, neck, and shoulder area, the flexors are used for elevation of the rib cage.

Develop a Breathing Rate of Less
Than 30 Cycles Per Minute

The kind of vocalizations from which speech develops requires prolonged exhalations of air which may be manipulated by the articulatory mechanism. Children whose rest-breathing pattern is characteristically rapid and shallow often have difficulty in producing prolonged exhalations. Among the possible causes of persistent rapid-breathing rates are that the child is incapable of the coordinated movements required for deeper breathing or that his posture prevents deeper inhalations. Procedures designed to break up tonic reflex patterns, facilitating developmental sequences leading to good sitting posture and maintenance of proper postural relationships between the neck and head, trunk and abdominal areas, seem to help certain cerebral palsied children achieve slower breathing rates.

Several procedures have been suggested for imposing a slower rest-breathing rate on the child. With the child lying on his back flex the knees and press the front portion of the upper legs against the abdomen by flexing the hips. Quickly extend the legs at the hips, thus releasing the pressure on the abdominal area. This pattern of movements should be repeated at a rate corresponding to the normal breathing rate, i.e., about 20 cycles per minute. A similar technique consists of crossing the child's forearms across his chest and pressing them tightly enough against his thorax to encourage a deeper exhalation. For inhalation, the pressure is released. The therapist times his movements of pressure and relaxation of pressure to correspond to the normal breathing pattern. Some therapists have the child breathe into a paper bag for a few minutes in an attempt to produce deeper and, hence, slower breathing. The rationale for this procedure is questionable. In rapid, shallow breathing, only the air in the top part of the lungs is changed. Alveolar air in the rest of the lung tends to become stagnant and consequently increases the carbon dioxide concentration in the blood. While normally carbon dioxide in the blood produces stimulation of the respiratory center in the central nervous system, an excess of carbon dioxide ceases to be a stimulant and concentrations of above 10 per cent may have an anesthetic effect. Techniques such as rebreathing, which are designed to increase the carbon dioxide concentration in the bloodstream, may have a place in the treatment of cerebral palsied children; but, they should not be used with those children who may already have a high carbon dioxide concentration.

Develop a Speech-Breathing Pattern of Quick Inhalation and Controlled, Prolonged Exhalation

Some cerebral palsied children, including those who have normal breathing rates, seem to have difficulty in learning to inhale quickly and then produce the controlled, prolonged exhalation required for continuous speech. Only in yawning or crying do these children have prolonged exhalations, and it is difficult to modify these breathing patterns for speech production. The first step in helping the child develop a speech-breathing pattern is to develop a quick inhalation. Momentary interference with inhalation—by holding a tissue over the nose and mouth—will cause the child to breathe deeply when the interference is removed. When carried out properly it is possible to use this technique even with small children. First occlude one nostril for a short period, *talking reassuringly* to the child as you do so. Next, occlude for a brief period both nostrils, forcing the child to breathe through his mouth. *Continue to talk reassuringly.* After the child is accustomed to this much interference with his breathing, cover the mouth also with the hand thus completely preventing breathing for a moment. Gradually increase the duration of the interference until a noticeably deep inhalation follows removal of the hand from the nose and mouth. It is helpful to hold a tissue in your hand and tell the child that you are going to put your hand over his nose and mouth just as if you were going to wipe his nose.

76   How do Rood (151: 220-24), Mysak (122), Westlake and Rutherford (189), Palmer (128: 514), and Mecham, Berko, and Berko (115) suggest teaching a child to develop a quick inhalation and a prolonged exhalation?

Producing deep inhalations on a reflex basis is only a first step. A child must next learn to hold the inhaled air until given a signal to exhale. At first the exhalations will be rapid and uncontrolled. Having the child imitate a prolonged sigh, a prolonged phonation, babbling, or sustained blowing will help him develop controlled, prolonged phonations. The child must also learn to produce the quick inhalation of adequate depth for speech on a voluntary basis. This seems to be easier for most children to learn after they have developed the ability to hold a reflex-induced inhalation and to produce a prolonged exhalation.

Counteract Abdominal Movements Which Are Asynchronous with Thoracic Movements

Sometimes cerebral palsy children are unable to produce prolonged exhalations because the abdominal-diaphragmatic movements are antagonistic to the thoracic movements. When this asynchrony is severe the child might be able to initiate a phonation or be able to produce only phonations of short duration. Some of these children are helped by a girdle which extends from the lower border of the sternum to below a line drawn between the crest of the ilia. This girdle should be a wraparound type made of duck material, with several strap and buckle combinations which permit sufficient tightening to restrict abdominal movements, thus permitting the thoracic movements to produce adequate inhalations and exhalations. For children with markedly asynchronous breathing patterns, girdles of this type often result in stronger voices and longer exhalations. Somewhat similar corsets are sometimes used to encourage abdominal expansion by limiting thoracic movement. In our experience, it seems to make little difference if the child's breathing pattern is predominantly abdominal or predominantly thoracic. The test of the adequacy of a breathing pattern is determined by the child's ability to inhale quickly and to produce a controlled, prolonged exhalation. Girdles or corsets should not be used indiscriminately with all cerebral palsy children who have breathing difficulties. In our opinion, they are indicated only in cases where asynchronous abdominal-thoracic movements interfere with the development of speech-breathing patterns and even then we are conservative in their use. They should be used only in a setting where the child is under close, frequent observation.

Functional Techniques for Developing Control of Respiration

Many techniques and pieces of equipment have been developed to encourage the child to produce prolonged exhalations. Usually these require sustained blowing, but some employ sustained phonations. Exercises requiring voluntary control of inhalation and exhalation are useful in developing speech-breathing patterns, but only when the child is ready for them. We have seen children whose improved blowing ability or increased durations of phonation could be dramatically demonstrated on a graph, but they were unable to use these increased exhalations in speech. Evaluation of their breathing patterns revealed marked asynchrony between the thoracic and abdominal muscle groups. Improvement in blowing and increase in duration of phonation had been achieved by increasing the tension in the abdominal muscles to squeeze the air out. Observation of the children revealed progressive increase in tension as phonation continued. Functional work with such interesting equipment as pin wheels, candles, spirometers, water bottles, and the like must be placed properly in the developmental sequences of breathing training.

> 77   Make a list of breathing training techniques suggested by various au-
>   thors. Describe the rationale for each in terms of the neurophysiology of
>   respiration and the types of breathing difficulties found in cerebral palsy.
>   Show where each would fit in the sequences of development of speech-
>   breathing skills. See Blumberg (13: 48-53), Cass (21), Gratke (70), Ruth-
>   erford (155).

IMPROVING PHONATION: PROBLEMS AND ILLUSTRATIVE TECHNIQUES

Laryngeal blocks occur as part of a more generalized pattern of neuromuscular dysfunction in cerebral palsied children; hence, any therapy designed to break up tonic reflex patterns, to achieve a more normal distribution of muscle tone, and to facilitate movement will contribute to the improvement of laryngeal function for speech. Also, laryngeal tension is related to the cerebral palsied child's speech-breathing pattern. When tension in the respiratory musculature increases as the child attempts to produce controlled, prolonged exhalations for speaking, the increased tension often spreads to the laryngeal musculature. Procedures for improving breathing patterns will also aid in developing adequate laryngeal function. In addition to these general approaches, the following more specific techniques are useful with children who have laryngeal dysfunction.

Encouraging Vocalization

Speech develops from sounds associated with feelings of pleasure rather than from crying sounds. Crying is useful to the cerebral palsied child in developing control of his larynx; he also learns that through his noise making he can exert some degree of control over his environment. Parents should learn not to respond to the crying so quickly that the child does not get sufficient practice in using his larynx or so slowly that he fails to appreciate the social utility of noise making.

Laughing also exercises the larynx; so, the cerebral palsied child should be encouraged to laugh. Gentle stroking or tickling over the ribs will produce the pattern of laryngeal action associated with reflex laughing. The mother should be encouraged to do this frequently as part of her play with the infant. Pleasurable vocalizing occurs most frequently after the child has been fed. A feeling of well being seems to be an adequate stimulus for this reflexive sound making. Parents should

> 78   At what times and under what circumstances is an infant most likely to vocalize? How can parents and therapists reinforce this early speech behavior? See Van Riper (*180*).

learn to enjoy their role of attentive members of the child's audience until he has finished his after-dinner vocal practice. When the child is about to stop, one of the parents should imitate the child's vocalizing to encourage him to continue. If a tape recorder is available for the family, some of the child's vocalizations might be recorded and then played back for the child in order to reinforce his sound-making efforts.

Because of severe breathing difficulties and/or laryngeal dysfunction some cerebral palsied children do little vocalizing. They are described by their parents as "quiet babies." Positioning is often useful in facilitating vocalization. The position in which vocalization is easiest varies from child to child. The following procedure is effective with many children. With the child in the supine position, place him in flexion, that is, with the head brought forward, the hands placed on opposite shoulders with the arms folded across the chest and the legs flexed at the knees and the hips. While holding the child in this position gently vibrate his sternum by pressing on it with the fingers and slowly rock him while making soft loving noises to him. Parents can be taught this technique as a way of playing with their child and should do it several times daily for short periods.

> 79   For a more detailed discussion of this procedure see Crickmay (*29*), Marland (*114:* 111-19) and Mysak (*122*).

Coordinate Phonation with Exhalation

After the child has learned to hold a deep inhalation until given a signal to exhale, he should be taught to phonate a vowel sound on the exhalation. Sometimes it is easier for the child to practice exhaling with an audible sigh before he learns to produce a phonation on the exhalation. If the child has difficulty initiating phonation, several different techniques for breaking up the laryngeal block should be tried. Gentle flexion and extension of the head and neck or slow turning of the head from side to side, either passively by the therapist or actively by the child, often produce variations in the tension of laryngeal muscles, thus permitting phonation. Positioning may also be used to good advantage. A child who has difficulty initiating phonation in the sitting position may be able to phonate more easily in a supine or prone position. Sometimes a child can start phonating if he is asked to imitate a higher or a lower pitch.

Develop Prolonged Phonations without Undesirable Tension

Speech therapists are often inclined to begin breathing training by instructing the cerebral palsy child to produce as long a phonation as he can and then, through the use of various motivating devices, encourage the child to longer and longer phonations. Before encouraging

80   How are chest and abdominal movements coordinated for the production and grouping of syllables? See McDonald (109) and Stetson (171).

the child to develop longer phonations, the therapist should be sure that the child inhales sufficiently immediately before beginning phonating. If a child tries to produce a long phonation on the air available in that part of the breathing cycle when he starts phonating, he is apt to become more and more tense as he struggles to produce a longer phonation. Also, the therapist should be sure that the child has learned to hold the inhaled air and to coordinate phonation with exhalation before attempting to develop long phonations.

After these preliminary skills have been developed, many techniques may be employed to develop controlled, prolonged phonations such as making a motor-like noise while "flying" a toy plane, keeping a graphic record of the duration of phonations, teaching the child to say a short phrase on one breath, or counting to some specified number on one breath. A general impression seems to have developed among speech therapists that a child should be able to phonate for at least ten seconds without interruption if the child is to be capable of producing connected speech. Sometimes other therapy, such as articulation training, is postponed until this goal is reached. Actually, most phrases spoken by normal adults are probably less than five seconds long. Easily initiated phonations are more important for speech production than long phonations. If, during a long phonation, a child builds up tension in the respiratory and laryngeal muscles, it will be more difficult for him to initiate the ensuing inhalation-exhalation cycle.

Develop Variations of Loudness and Pitch

Practice in producing tones at different levels of loudness, with different inflection patterns, and at different pitch levels will help the child increase his control of laryngeal function. Only a little imagination is required to think of many ways to motivate the child to vary the loudness, pitch, or inflection patterns of his voice. Role-playing activities in which the child pretends he is whispering a secret, or giving an order like the corner policeman, or cheering at a sports event, and so forth are effective. Singing works well with children of nursery-school age and above. Children's attention might be directed to the kind of voice they use when saying their prayers or mealtime grace, when calling a parent or someone from another room, and when talking to someone nearby.

Counteract Undesirable Postural Patterns

During speech therapy, the therapist should be watching for postural patterns which seem to interfere with laryngeal function. One of the most common is an extensor thrust which seems to accompany attempts at phonation in some children. As the child phonates he will be seen to extend the legs, arch the back, and throw back his head. In some cases this will be extreme and readily noticeable. In other cases the generalized increase in extensor tone will produce only slight movements. These can be detected by placing one's hand against the soles of the child's feet, on his shoulders, or behind his head. The speech therapist must learn how to feel these changes in flexor and extensor tone. When increases in extensor tone are associated with phonation, consideration should be given to using appropriate reflex-inhibiting postures or appropriate sensory stimulation for activation and inhibition of selected muscle groups. These techniques the speech therapist must learn by studying with someone who is properly trained in using the techniques. If the child is using a relaxation chair, jack-knifing the seat causing flexion at the hips will often break up the extensor thrust.

There is another pattern which is often seen in cerebral palsied children. When they extend their necks to bring the head into an upright position, they often throw the chin upward and forward. This movement is sometimes encouraged by feeding practices in which the feeder's hand is placed under the child's chin and the chin pulled forward and upward before the food is put into the child's mouth. For children with adequate breathing patterns and no laryngeal involvement this maneuver does not interfere with speech production. When adequate laryngeal control has not been developed, this maneuver sometimes seems to trigger laryngeal spasms.

> 81   Make a list of the various techniques which have been suggested for improving phonation. Describe the rationale for each technique in terms of the neurophysiology of phonation and the kinds of laryngeal involvement found in cerebral palsy. Determine at what stage of training the various techniques might be applicable. See Palmer (131: 40-41), Rutherford (155), Gratke (70), Cass (21), Mecham, Berko, and Berko (115).

TRAINING IN ARTICULATION: PROBLEMS AND ILLUSTRATIVE TECHNIQUES

Viewed as one of the processes by which speech is produced, articulation consists of temporally overlapping movements of the articulatory structures, particularly the lips, tongue, and mandible. These movements create obstructions of varying degree and location in the path of the exhaled air. Before it is influenced by the interrelated processes of articulation and resonation, the airstream may already have been modified by the process of phonation. It is obvious that the child must first develop adequate control of his respiratory and laryngeal functions before he can master articulatory skills. While, in treating cerebral palsied children, some aspects of the training in articulation, phonation, and respiration can go on simultaneously, *therapists should be sure that the child has sufficient| control over speech breathing and phonation.* Also, there are patterns of neural organization of the articulatory function, such as those used in sucking and swallowing, which must be developed before a child can develop efficient use of his articulatory mechanism for the production of speech sounds.

Encourage and Facilitate Babbling

The earliest vocalizations of the infant consist of prolonged vowels, but soon random movement of the articulators modifies the vowel sounds into consonant-vowel combinations. It has been frequently pointed out that during his first year the normal child will have babbled many times all the speech sounds he will use later in his life. Even deaf infants start babbling at an early age and continue to do so for several months in much the same way as do normal children. Many cerebral palsied children, however, do not babble or babble only in a limited way by practicing just a few sounds. Babbling is so essential to the later development of mature articulation skills that parents of silent cerebral palsied infants should be taught how to facilitate babbling. While an infant is crying, it is sometimes possible to effect approximation of the lips by placing the hand beneath the mandible and gently elevating it. Repetition of this maneuver enables the child to hear and feel the consonantal modification of his vocalization.

In an earlier section we described how to facilitate vocalizing with the child flexed in the supine position. After the child has begun to produce lengthy vocalizations in this position, bilabial consonants may be added by rapidly vibrating the lips with the therapist's or parent's fingers. To capitalize on the child's natural tendency for vocal play and other motor activity following a meal and at other comfortable moments in his life, a large mirror might be suspended above his bed to add visual stimulation and reinforcement for his babbling efforts. Again, when he seems about to stop babbling his parents should be ready to stimulate the child with imitations of his babbling.

Develop Sucking, Swallowing, and Chewing Patterns

At birth, the neonate has several reflexes associated with sucking which seem to operate to bring the infant's mouth into contact with the nipple and to position the lips for sucking. Drooling occurs during sucking because lip movements are not well coordinated with tongue movements and control of the corners of the lips has not yet developed. Swallowing reflexes are also present at birth; however, the oral stage of swallowing, which is a voluntary stage, is poorly developed. Coordination of many muscle groups must be developed to produce the lip closure, elevation of the mandible, elevation of the soft palate, and proper timing of movements of different parts of the tongue which comprise the voluntary stage of swallowing. Biting reflexes are present, but chewing patterns are not included in the neuromuscular organization of the neonate. In the normal child, primitive sucking, swallowing, and chewing patterns are modified through maturation and learning. Many cerebral palsied children do not progress beyond the infantile stages without help.

> 82 What is the sequence of development of sucking, swallowing, and chewing skills. See Gesell (64). What infantile reflexes may interfere with this development? See Mysak (124: 252-60).

Attention should be given to the development of sucking, swallowing, and chewing patterns in cerebral palsied children as soon as possible. As a part of her feeding routine, the mother can use a number of techniques which will facilitate maturation of oral activities. Since these children are often difficult to feed, the tendency is to do it in the easiest way for the mother and to get it over with as quickly as possible. Actually it is beneficial for the child to have even more opportunities to practice sucking and swallowing than it is for the normal child. In fact, his mother should prolong feeding by touching the nipple to his lips to tease him into making sucking movements and by using feeding methods which, while they require more time, will strengthen muscles which will later be used for articulating. For example, rather than always holding the child in a position which allows gravity to carry the milk back into his throat, she should use other positions which will make the child work harder to suck and swallow. Stimulation of reflexes is important. Particularly during the early part of the feeding period while the child is hungry, the mother should stimulate the lip reflex by tapping near the angle of the mouth and the sucking reflex by placing her finger or a nipple in contact with the lips and front of the tongue. Periodically throughout the day, the mother should stimulate lip and suckling reflexes.

When spooned foods are added to the child's diet, care should be exercised to place the food in the front of the mouth, thus encouraging the child to develop the tongue movements which are essential for the first stage of chewing and the first stage of swallowing. Touching the child's lips with the spoon will heighten his awareness of his lips and thus facilitate the maintenance of lip closure.

83   Do Westlake's suggestions for modified feeding (*188*) and Palmer's techniques for normalizing chewing, sucking, and swallowing reflexes (*132: 415-18*) have similar rationales?

While with infants it may be necessary to stimulate infantile reflex patterns, unless these eventually drop out, it will be necessary to break up the persistent infantile patterns of the older child. Of all the reflexes listed on page 123 which involve structures used in articulating, the persistent suckling, biting, and lip reflexes are most likely to interfere with developing mature sucking, swallowing, chewing, and articulatory activities. Two methods are effective in breaking up persistent infantile patterns in the older cerebral palsied child. One consists of applying the appropriate stimulus for the reflex and then inhibiting its response. For example, the corner of the lips might be tapped to stimu-

REFLEXES INVOLVING STRUCTURES
WHICH ARE USED IN ARTICULATION

Name	Stimulus	Response
Cephalic reactions	Stroking the lobe of the ear or the nostril	Turns head away from stimulus
Facial response	Sharp tapping around mouth	Rounding and protrusion of lips as in pouting
Rooting reflex	Repeated light stroking of the cheek or around the mouth	Movement of the head as if trying to get a nipple into the mouth
Mouth opening	Sight of an object such as a nipple, finger, or tongue depressor, which is usually associated with mouth opening	Lowering of mandible and separation of lips
Lip reflex	Tapping around the angle formed at the corner of the mouth	Involuntary movements of the lips— lip closure and pouting
Biting reflex	Object placed between teeth (or gums)	Strong, sustained elevation of mandible
Suckling reflex	Gentle pushing and pulling on a nipple or finger placed in mouth	Alternating protruding and retracting movements of the tongue often with elevation of the tip
Chewing reflex	Tapping the teeth or gums with a tongue blade	Alternating elevations and depressions of the mandible
Laughing	Light stroking or tickling particularly of the sides of the thorax	Involuntary twitching of the body, opening of mouth, disruption of breathing rhythm, often accompanied by sound production on both inhalation and exhalation
Swallowing Oral stage (Voluntary)	Presence of food or liquid in oral cavity	Wavelike motion of tongue to propel food into oropharynx
Pharyngeal stage (Reflex)	Contact of food or fluid with mucosa of faucial pillars and pharyngeal wall	Contraction of faucial pillars and walls of pharynx, elevation of palate, elevation and closing of larynx and momentary suspension of respiration

late the lip reflex and then the lips held with the fingers to prevent the involuntary motions of the reflex. Another technique is to present one or more stimuli simultaneously with the appropriate stimuli and in that way weaken the stimulus-response bond. For example, while tapping the corners of the mouth to elicit the lip reflex, the cheek might be patted, the gums gently rubbed, or the mandible moved up and down gently.

Many suggestions are available to the therapist for improving sucking, swallowing, and chewing patterns. These emphasize modified feeding techniques and methods for teaching straw drinking. These procedures are valuable but should not be used until the child's problem has been carefully analyzed and careful consideration is given to where these techniques fit into the maturational sequences.

Improving the Function of the Lips, Mandible, and Tongue as Articulators

The articulatory use of the oral structures varies in many ways from the more gross vegetative functions. Articulatory movements are more rapid, must be more precisely integrated with activities of other muscle systems, give rise to more selective sensory stimulations, and use a different selection of the available movements. For example, elevation of the tongue tip is common in articulation, but lateralization of the tongue tip is more common in vegetative function. Of particular importance in articulating is the ability to disassociate movements of the tongue from movements of the mandible or lip. The therapist should help the child heighten his awareness of the movement of the various articulators. By watching himself in a mirror, the child can see that his mandible moves with his tongue movements. Encouraging exaggeration of the undesirable movement will make it more obvious to the child. Stabilization of the mandible with a small object, such as a piece of a stiff eraser placed between the molars, aids the child in developing free tongue movements.

> 84   How would you use negative practice, see Rutherford (154: 259-64), resistance, see Hoberman (82: 111-23), and passive manipulation, see Cass (21), in developing lip, tongue, and jaw movements?

Improving diadochokinetic actions of the structures is an important step in the articulation training program, but it is to be remembered that the movements of articulation are characteristically rapid and overlapping. To develop ability to produce the overlapping movements of articulation, the child should be given practice with syllables containing phonetic contexts which will elicit desired overlapping patterns of movement. For example, in the bisyllable *up da,* which a child might say when he wants his father to pick him up, the tip of the tongue is elevating for [d] while the lips are approximated for [p]. In *hit me,* the lips close for [m] while the tip of the tongue is elevated for [t]. In the first words of a child and in most of his jargon, consonants are usually preceded and followed by a vowel. As soon as he begins making two-word sentences, intersyllabic consonantal adjacencies (*abutting consonants*) occur. Later, consonantal adjacencies (called *compound consonants* or *blends*) occur within a syllable. Drill only with consonant-vowel combinations, such as *ma ma, da da, baby,* does not develop the complex overlapping movements which occur in the production of abutting and compound consonants. Speech therapy should include practice with bisyllables containing abutting consonants requiring overlapping movements of the lips and tongue and later with abutting consonants requiring overlapping movements within the tongue.

MOTIVATING THE CHILD TO TALK

Speech therapists have long been skillful in developing motivational devices. Puppets, gadgets, card games, and many other devices have been described for motivating the speech-defective child to practice what the therapist has planned for the therapy session. These techniques are often useful, but reliance on them leads to only superficial and temporary motivation. Greater attention should be given to basic psychosocial needs which contribute to the formation of deeper and longer-lasting motivations.

Desire to Become Self-Determining

Almost from birth one can observe the normal infant struggling to establish an independent existence. Constantly the child tries to assume greater and greater power in making decisions about those matters which will have an influence on him as an individual. The normal child soon learns that he can effectively announce his decisions by uttering the monosyllables *yes* or *no* and is motivated to increase his potential for self-determination by learning and using more language and speech. The ability to move about freely brings many opportunities for decision making to a normal child.

What about the cerebral palsied child? Normal children have to fight for opportunities to fulfill their need to become independent. To adults, children always seem unprepared for making decisions. With what weapons can the severely involved cerebral palsied child fight? Because he is physically disabled, he can't run away or strike out. If he has not developed speech, he can't lash out verbally at those who make all his decisions for him.

Parents and therapists should constantly be alert for ways to help the cerebral palsied child become self-assertive. Early use of questions which require the child to make a choice encourages him to use speech. For example, a mother might ask a young child, "Do you want your doll or your bunny?" Or a father might ask, "Do you want to get into your pajamas first or have your teeth brushed first?" When parents become aware of how important it is for their cerebral palsied child to learn to think of himself as an individual, they will devise many ways to strengthen his self-concept and, thus, increase his motivation to talk. Above all parents must be helped to realize that overprotection robs their child of opportunities to become independent.

Need for Social Relationships

Even while the normal child is striving to establish his independence he desires the company of other people. Actually, the normal child acquires a sense of other selves before he acquires a clear sense of his own self. The child's first personal-social relations revolve mainly around persons older than himself. However, beginning at an early age he becomes increasingly involved in a society of his peers. Fulfillment of his need for social acceptance is sought more and more from the peer group as he grows older and there is a concurrent reduction in his need for approval from his family. Speech is one of the child's basic tools for interrelating with his peers.

Again, what about the cerebral palsied child? His interactions with other people, adults and peers, differ from those of normal children in both quantity and quality. During childhood the cerebral palsied child's social interactions are dominated by adults who study, treat, or teach him. The peer relationship of severely handicapped cerebral palsied children are markedly restricted. His need for social relationships is largely unfulfilled, and the motivation for speech and language use which naturally results from peer interaction remains undeveloped.

Every effort should be made to provide early and continuing opportunities for the severely involved cerebral palsied child to interact with a peer group. Regularly scheduled group meetings stressing social-ization activities should be included in the rehabilitation program of the young cerebral palsied child. Speech therapy should stress efforts to motivate the child through planned opportunities for social interaction with peers rather than to provide only opportunities for the child to relate to an adult therapist.

85 How can language and speech activities be integrated into preschool training programs for cerebral palsied children? See Gillette (65: 31-34), Plotkin (147: 16-20), and (149).

HELPING THE OLDER CHILD AND ADOLESCENT

It is not to be expected that early application of available principles and methods of language and speech therapy will produce normal speech for all cerebral palsied persons. Even the most conscientious efforts of therapists and patients will sometimes fail to develop the specificity of sensory-motor function essential to the production of even intelligible speech. In many cases usable but defective speech will represent the outcome of many years of therapy. Following are some procedures which may be effective in improving the oral com-munication skills of the older cerebral palsied child or adolescent.

Heighten the Patient's Desire to Make Himself Understood

Parents and close associates often learn to interpret with relative ease the defective and minimal communication efforts of the cerebral palsied child: consequently, the child does not make an effective effort to make himself understood. Unless the cerebral palsied individual is sufficiently concerned about making himself understood by persons outside his close circle of acquaintances, all efforts to improve his speech will be futile.

Help the Patient Find a Method of Self-Stabilization

At times the intelligibility of speech is reduced by gross involuntary movements in the upper part of the body which accompany efforts at speech production. Many cerebral palsied persons independently de-velop effective methods of controlling or reducing these involuntary movements. For example, some patients may be observed to wedge a hard-to-control arm between their body and the arm of a wheelchair. Others develop the habit of sitting on their hand to control the involuntary movements of an arm.

Teach Patients to Limit Phrase Length to That Portion of an Exhalation Which Can Be Produced without Increase in Tension

A common trigger of tension or involuntary movement in adolescents is the effort made to continue talking when there is insufficient air for speech production. Often their speech is intelligible at the beginning of the phrase but becomes weak and difficult to understand near the end of a phrase of even six or seven syllables. The therapist should try to determine an optimal phrase length for each individual and to train the patient to limit phrases to the optimal length.

Develop Variety in the Rate, Pitch, and Intensity of Speech

The speech of some cerebral palsied individuals is extremely monotonous. Therapy sessions in which the patient is taught to analyze the inflection patterns of normal speech and is given guidance in imitating normal inflection patterns is sometimes helpful.

Help the Patient Learn to Relax the Tension Which Develops during Speech Attempts

We have never been very successful in employing relaxation techniques to counteract the primary tension characteristic of several types of cerebral palsy. In addition to this tension, however, adolescents often exhibit secondary tensions which have become associated with speaking. These secondary tensions can often be eliminated through analysis, negative practice and conscious control. Similar methods are sometimes helpful in reducing the grimacing associated with speaking.

Help Close Associates of the Patient Understand his Problems

When an associate fails to understand the cerebral palsied person's problems or is insensitive to his feelings, communication often deteriorates. We once saw a severely involved thirty-year-old spastic quadriplegic female whose frequent regurgitations made her difficult to feed. For years her mother thought sheer stubbornness prompted the daughter to spit out the food, and the relationship between the mother and daughter was constantly strained. Their communication was forced and unpleasant. When we were able to demonstrate that strong spasms in the pharyngeal muscles prevented swallowing and forced the food back into her mouth, both mother and daughter were appreciative. One of the common attitudes to be counteracted is that the cerebral palsied person could do better "if he only tried."

When the Patient Is Unable to Develop Socially Useful Oral Communication Skills, Assist Him to Develop a Personalized Conversation or Language Board

There will be occasions when objective assessment of the cerebral palsied child's problems indicates that despite good intellectual potential, normal hearing, and adequately developed language concepts, it will be impossible to develop usable oral communication skills. Continued efforts to develop speech lead only to frustration of the patient and the therapist. Yet the patient feels equally frustrated by his inability to express himself in any way. Two devices may reduce the patient's frustrations.

Identification Cards

An older patient who cannot make himself understood to anyone but his immediate family often lives in fear that he may someday find it necessary to communicate when no member of his family is available. A teen-ager, for example, became extemely frightened and insecure when his mother was injured in an automobile accident while taking him to a clinic. He wanted to carry a set of cards bearing his name, describing his condition, giving his home address, father's business address, etc. Some adolescents want questions about basic needs on the cards so that they can nod yes or no when shown the card.

Language Boards

Communication devices of varying complexity may be developed for use as a teaching tool or for carrying on conversations. In developing a language board, it is essential that the child participate in organizing it. Words or symbols of the child's choosing should be used in the first simple form of the board. Depending on the child's intellectual ability, language units of increasing complexity should be employed in successive boards.

86 How would you develop a language board for a child of kindergarten level? Of primary-grade level? A conversation board for an adolescent? See Goldberg and Fenton (68).

🎵🎵🎵

Have we enough information to do some tentative planning of speech programs for the group of cerebral palsied children introduced in Chapter I? Charles Pounka presents us with an interesting problem. He's the boy who writes with his feet. He understands language, but it is difficult for him to initiate vocalizations. That observation plus the notes concerning the presence of a persistent tonic neck reflex and poor control of the upper extremities are suggestive of both a laryngeal block and an inadequate speech-breathing pattern. Does he need language stimulation? Is he ready for articulation training? What would you try first with Charles if you were his therapist? Let's suppose that Clayton Penths, Charleen Pimskon, Catherine Pombst, Carl Pednok, and Clifford Puzin also were enrolled in your clinic. Would you schedule them for speech therapy? What would your preliminary plan be for each?

Even this practice planning for our small group of cerebral palsied children emphasizes our point that there is no ready-made, sure-fire method of speech therapy for cerebral palsy. The program for each child must be designed individually to meet *his* special needs. Again we want to emphasize that the treatment procedures described in this chapter are intended to be illustrative. Many more have been described by other authors and the creative therapist will create many of his own. Too often, however, methods are created or applied with little reference to the principles which should underlie sound treatment procedures. Methods should derive from principles. This is not to say that principles are important while methods are unimportant. Clinical competence consists not only of knowing what to do in the long run, but also of knowing what to do *now*. Principles help determine what to do in the long run; methods which are based on principles tell the therapist what to do *now*. The complex habilitation problems of the cerebral palsied child will challenge the ingenuity of the therapist to discover new principles and to develop new methods. There remain many still to be discovered. 🎵🎵🎵

bibliography

1. Aird, R. B.,and P. Cohen, "Electroencephalography in Cerebral Palsy," *Journal of Pediatrics*, XXXVII (1950).
2. Allen, R. M., and T. W. Jefferson, *Psychological Evaluation of the Cerebral Palsied Person* (Springfield, Ill.: Charles C Thomas, Publisher, 1962).
3. Altman, I., "On the Prevalence of Cerebral Palsy," *Cerebral Palsy Review*, XVI (1955).
4. Anderson, G. W., "Current Needs for Research on the Obstetrical Factors in Cerebral Palsy," *Cerebral Palsy Review*, XIV (1953).
5. Asher, P., "A Study of 63 Cases of Athetosis with Special Reference to Hearing Defects," *Archives of Disease in Childhood*, XXVII (1952).
6. Ayres, A. J., "Occupational Therapy for Motor Disorders Resulting from Impairment of the Central Nervous System." *Rehabilitation Literature*, XXI (1960).
7. Barry, H., *The Young Aphasic Child: Evaluation and Training* (Washington, D. C.: The Alexander Graham Bell Association for the Deaf, Inc., 1961).
8. Bender, L., and A. Silver, "Body Image Problems in the Brain Damaged Child," *The Journal of Social Issues*, IV (1948).

9. Berenberg, W., R. Byers, and E. Meyers, "Cerebral Palsy Nursery Schools," *Quarterly Review of Pediatrics,* VII (1952).
10. Bexton, W. H., W. Heron, and T. H. Scott, "Effects of Decreased Variation in the Sensory Environment," *Canadian Journal of Psychology,* VIII (1954).
11. Bice, H. V., *Group Counseling of Mothers of the Cerebral Palsied,* (Chicago: The National Society for Crippled Children and Adults, 1952).
12. ———, "Some Factors that Contribute to the Concept of Self in the Child with Cerebral Palsy," *Mental Hygiene,* XXXVIII (1954).
ᐟ13. Blumberg, M. L., "Respiration and Speech in the Cerebral Palsied Child," *American Journal of Diseases of Children,* XXCIX (1955).
14. Bobath, B., "The Treatment of Motor Disorders of Pyramidal and Extrapyramidal Origin by Reflex Inhibition and by Facilitation of Movements," *Physiotherapy,* XLI (1955).
15. Bobath, K. and B. Bobath, "Tonic Neck Reflexes and Righting Reflexes in Diagnosis and Assessment of Cerebral Palsy," *Cerebral Palsy Review,* XVI (1955).
16. ———, and ———, "Treatment of Cerebral Palsy Based on Analysis of Patients' Motor Behavior," *British Journal of Physical Medicine,* XV (1952).
17. Bobath, B., and K. Bobath, "Treatment of Cerebral Palsy by the Inhibition of Abnormal Reflex Action," *British Orthoptic Journal,* XI (1954).
18. Bruner, J. S., "The Course of Cognitive Growth," *American Psychologist,* XIX (1964).
19. Byers, R. K., R. S. Paine, and B. Crothers, "Extrapyramidal Cerebral Palsy with Hearing Loss Following Erythroblastosis," *Pediatrics,* XV (1955).
20. Cardwell, V., *Cerebral Palsy: Advances in Understanding and Care,* (New York: Association for the Aid of Crippled Children, 1956).
21. Cass, M. T., *Speech Habilitation in Cerebral Palsy* (New York: Columbia University Press, 1951).
22. *Cerebral Palsy Equipment,* (Chicago: National Society for Crippled Children and Adults, 1953).
23. Chusid, J. G., and J. J. McDonald, *Correlative Neuroanatomy and Functional Neurology,* 11th ed. (Los Altos, Calif.: Lange Medical Publications, 1962).
24. Collaborative Perinatal Research Project: 5 Years of Progress, *Collaborative Project Reporter,* National Institute Neurological Disorders and Blindness, Special Issue, Autumn 1963.
25. Collis, E., "Management of Cerebral Palsy in Children," *Medicine Illustrated,* VII (1953).
26. ———, *A Way of Life for the Handicapped Child: A New Approach to Cerebral Palsy* (London: Faber and Faber, Ltd., 1947).
27. ———, "Results of Treatment of Infantile Cerebral Palsy," *Lancet,* I. (1953).
28. Courville, C. B., *Cerebral Palsy* (Los Angeles: San Lucas Press, 1954).
29. Crickmay, M., *Description and Orientation of the Bobath Method*

with Reference to Speech Rehabilitation in Cerebral Palsy (Chicago: National Society for Crippled Children and Adults, 1956).

30. Cruickshank, W., and J. Dolphin, "Educational Implications of Psychological Studies of Cerebral Palsied Children," *Exceptional Children,* XVIII (1951).

31. ————, H. Bice and N. Wallen, *Perception and Cerebral Palsy* (Syracuse: Syracuse University Press, 1957).

32. ————, and G. M. Raus, *Cerebral Palsy: Its Individual and Community Problems* (Syracuse: Syracuse University Press, 1955).

33. Curran, P. A., "A Study toward a Theory of Neuromuscular Education through Occupational Therapy," *American Journal of Occupational Therapy,* XIV (1960).

34. Darley, F. A., ed., *Symposium on Cerebral Palsy* (Washington, D. C.: American Speech and Hearing Association, 1962).

35. ————, *Diagnosis and Appraisal of Communication Disorders* (Englewood Cliffs, N. J.: Prentice-Hall, Inc., 1964).

36. Deaver, G., "Etiological Factors in Cerebral Palsy," *Bulletin of New York Academy of Medicine,* XXVIII (1952).

37. ————, *Cerebral Palsy: Methods of Evaluation and Treatment,* Rehabilitation Monograph IX (New York: Institute of Physical Medicine and Rehabilitation, 1955).

38. ————, "Cerebral Palsy: Methods of Treating Neuromuscular Disabilities," *Archives of Physical Medicine and Rehabilitation,* XXXVII (1956).

39. De Jong, R. N., *Neurologic Examination* (New York: Paul B. Hoeber, 1958).

40. Denhoff, E., "A Primer of Cerebral Palsy for the General Practitioner," *Medical Times* (April 1953). Reprinted by the National Society for Crippled Children and Adults, Chicago.

41. ————, and R. Holden, "Family Influence on Successful School Adjustment of Cerebral Palsied Children," *Exceptional Children,* XXI (1954).

42. ————, and ————, "Significance of Delayed Development in the Diagnosis of Cerebral Palsy," *Journal of Pediatrics,* XXXVIII (1951).

43. ———— and I. Robinault, *Cerebral Palsy and Related Disorders* (New York: McGraw-Hill Book Company, 1960).

44. Denny-Brown, D., "Motor Mechanisms—Introduction: The General Principles of Motor Integration," in *Handbook of Physiology,* ed. J. Field, Section 1: Neurophysiology (Washington, D. C.: American Physiological Society, 1960) II.

45. Dick, A. P. and C. J. Stevenson, "Hereditary Spastic Paraplegia, Report of a Family with Associated Extrapyramidal Signs," *Lancet,* CCLXIV (1953).

46. Doll, E. A., *Measurement of Social Competence* (New York: Educational Publishers, Inc., 1953).

47. Dunsdon, M. I., *The Educability of Cerebral Palsied Children* (London: Newnes Educational Publishing Co. Ltd., 1952).

48. Duvall, N. E., *Kinesiology: The Anatomy of Motion,* (Englewood Cliffs, N. J.: Prentice-Hall, Inc., 1959).

49. Egel, P., *Technique of Treatment for the Cerebral Palsied Child* (St. Louis: C. V. Mosby Co., 1948).

50. *Epilepsy—The Ghost Is Out of the Closet,* Public Affairs Pamphlet No. 98 (New York: Public Affairs Committee, Inc., 1945).

51. Evans, P. R., "Antecedents of Infantile Cerebral Palsy," *Archives of Diseases of Childhood,* XXIII (1948).

52. Fairbanks, G., "A Theory of the Speech Mechanism as a Servosystem," *Journal of Speech and Hearing Disorders,* XIX (1954).

53. Fay, T., "Rehabilitation of Patients with Spastic Paralysis," *Journal of International College of Surgeons,* XXII (1954).

54. ———, "The Neurophysical Aspects of Therapy in Cerebral Palsy," *Archives of Physical Medicine,* XXIX (1948).

55. ———, "The Origin of Human Movement," *American Journal of Psychiatry,* III (1955).

56. ———, "Use of Pathological and Unlocking Reflexes," *American Journal of Physical Medicine,* XXXIII (1954).

57. Fisch, L., "Deafness in Cerebral Palsied School Children," *Lancet,* II (1955).

58. Fishbein, M., ed., *Birth Defects,* (Philadelphia: J. B. Lippincott Company, 1963).

59. Fisher, S. and S. E. Cleveland, *Body Image and Personality* (New York: Van Nostrand, 1958).

60. Fulton, J. F., *Physiology of the Nervous System,* 3rd ed., (New York: Oxford University Press, 1949).

61. Gardner, E., *Fundamentals of Neurology,* 2nd ed. (Philadelphia: W. B. Saunders Company, 1958).

62. Garmezy, N., "Some Problems for Psychological Research in Cerebral Palsy," *American Journal of Physical Medicine* XXXII (1953).

63. Gesell, A., *The First Five Years of Life* (New York: Harper & Row, Publishers, Inc., 1940).

64. ———, and F. Ilg, *Feeding Behavior of Infants* (Philadelphia: J. B. Lippincott Company, 1937).

65. Gillette, H., "Preschool Training for Cerebral Palsy," *Archives of Physical Medicine and Rehabilitation,* XXXVI (1955).

66. ———, "The Treatment of Cerebral Palsy," *Physical Therapy Review,* XXXII (1952).

67. Ginsburg, M. M., "Congenital Spastic Paralysis Occurring in Four Members of One Family," *Rocky Mountain Medical Journal,* XXXVI (1939).

68. Goldberg, H. R., and J. Fenton, eds., *Aphonic Communication for Those with Cerebral Palsy,* (New York: United Cerebral Palsy Associations of New York, n.d.).

69. Granit, R., *Receptors and Sensory Perception,* (New Haven: Yale University Press, 1955).

70. Gratke, J. M., *Help Them Help Themselves* (Dallas: Texas Society for Crippled Children, 1947).

71. Grayson, J., *Nerves, Brain and Man* (New York: Taplinger Publishing Co. Inc., 1960).

72. Greenspan, L., and G. Deaver, "Clinical Approach to Etiologic Factors

in Cerebral Palsy," *Archives of Physical Medicine and Rehabilitation,* XXXIV (1953).

73. Guibor, G. P., "A Practical Routine for Discerning Oculomotor Defects in Cerebral Palsied Children," *Journal of Pediatrics,* XLIX (1955).

74. ———, "Some Eye Defects Seen in Cerebral Palsy with Some Statistics," *Archives of Ophthalmology,* LV (1955).

75. Hanna, R., "The Function of a Cerebral Palsy Treatment Center," *Cerebral Palsy Review,* XVI (1955).

76. Hardy, J. C., "Intraoral Breath Pressure in Cerebral Palsy," *Journal of Speech and Hearing Disorders,* XXVI (1961).

77. Hardy, W. G., "Hearing Impairment in Cerebral Palsied Children," *Cerebral Palsy Review,* XIV (1953).

78. Hastings, R., "Bracing for Cerebral Palsy," *Physical Therapy Review,* XXVIII (1950).

79. Haussermann, E., "Evaluating the Developmental Level of Cerebral Palsy Preschool Children," *Journal of Genetic Psychology,* XXC (1952).

80. Hebb, D. O., "The Motivating Effects of Exteroceptive Stimulation," *American Psychologist,* XIII (1958).

81. Hellebrandt, F. A., "The Physiology of Motor Learning," *Cerebral Palsy Review* (July-August 1958).

82. Hoberman, S. E., and M. Hoberman, "Speech Rehabilitation in Cerebral Palsy," *Journal of Speech and Hearing Disorders* XXV (1960).

83. Hohman, L., L. Baker, and R. Reed, "Sensory Disturbances in Children with Infantile Hemiplegia, Triplegia and Quadriplegia," *American Journal of Physical Medicine,* XXXVII (1958).

84. Hopkins, T. H., H. V. Bice, and M. Cotton, *Evaluation and Education of the Cerebral Palsied Child* (Washington, D. C.: International Council for Exceptional Children, 1954).

85. Hughes, R. R., *An Introduction to Clinical Electroencephalography* (Baltimore: Williams and Wilkins, 1961).

86. Hull, H. C., "Study of the Respiration of Fourteen Spastic Paralysis Cases during Silence and Speech," *Journal of Speech Disorders,* V (1940).

87. Hunt, J. McV., *Intelligence and Experience* (New York: The Ronald Press Co., 1961).

88. Ilg, F. M., and L. B. Ames, *Child Behavior* (New York: Dell Publishing Co., 1955).

89. Illingworth, R. S., ed., *Cerebral Palsy* (Boston: Little, Brown & Co., 1958).

90. Ingram, T. T. S., "A Study of Cerebral Palsy in the Childhood Population of Edinburg," *Archives of Diseases of Children,* XXX (1955).

91. Irwin, O. C. and H. P. Chen, "Speech Sound Elements during the First Year of Life: A Review of the Literature," *Journal of Speech Disorders,* VIII (1943).

92. Johnson, W., F. Darley, and D. Spriestersbach, *Diagnostic Methods in Speech Pathology* (New York: Harper & Row, Publishers, Inc., 1963).

93. Kabat, H., "Proprioceptive Facilitation in Therapeutic Exercise," in *Therapeutic Exercise, Physical Medicine Library*, ed. S. Licht (Baltimore: Waverley Press, 1958).

94. ———, "Central Facilitation: the Basis of Treatment for Paralysis," *Permanente Foundation Medical Bulletin*, X (1952).

95. ———, "Central Mechanisms for Recovery of Neuromuscular Function," *Science*, CXII (1950).

96. Kaplan, H. M., *Anatomy and Physiology of Speech* (New York: McGraw-Hill Book Company, 1960).

97. Kastein, S., "Speech Therapy in Cerebral Palsy," *Journal of Rehabilitation*, XIV (1948).

98. ———, "Speech Hygiene Guidance for Parents with C. P. Children," *Cerebral Palsy Review* (November 1950).

99. Keith, H. M., M. A. Norval, and A. B. Hunt, "Neurologic Lesions in the Newly Born Infant," *Pediatrics*, VI (1950).

100. Kirk, S. A. and J. J. McCarthy, "The Illinois Test of Psycholinguistic Abilities—An Approach to Differential Diagnosis," *American Journal of Mental Deficiency*, LXVI (1961).

101. Knott, M., "Specialized Neuromuscular Techniques in the Treatment of Cerebral Palsy," *Physical Therapy Review*, XXXII (1952).

102. ———, and D. E. Voss, *Proprioceptive Neuromuscular Facilitation: Patterns and Techniques* (New York: Paul B. Hoeber, Inc., 1956).

103. Koven, M. T., "Braces and Bracing," *Cerebral Palsy Review*, XV (1954).

104. Lefevre, M. C., "A Rationale for Resistive Therapy in Speech Training for the Cerebral Palsied," *Exceptional Children*, XIX (1952).

105. Levinson, H., "A Parent Training Program for a Cerebral Palsy Unit," *Journal of Speech and Hearing Disorders*, XIX (1954).

106. Lillywhite, H., "Make Mother a Clinician," *Journal of Speech and Hearing Disorders*, XIII (1948).

107. Little, W. J., "On the Influence of Abnormal Parturition, Difficult Labours, Premature Birth, and Asphyxia Neonatorum on the Mental and Physical Condition of the Child, Especially in Relation to Deformities, *Lancet*, II (1861).

108. McDonald, E. T., *Understand Those Feelings: A Guide for Parents of Handicapped Children and Everyone Who Counsels Them* (Pittsburgh: Stanwix House, Inc., 1962).

109. ———, *Articulation Testing and Treatment: A Sensory-Motor Approach* (Pittsburgh, Stanwix House, Inc., 1964).

110. McGinnis, M. A., *Aphasic Children: Identification and Education by the Association Method* (Washington, D. C.: Alexander Graham Bell Association for the Deaf, 1963).

111. Magoun, H. W., *The Waking Brain*, 2nd ed. (Springfield: Charles C Thomas, Publisher, 1963).

112. ———, "Physiology of the Cerebral Cortex and Basal Ganglia in Relation to the Symptoms of Cerebral Palsy," *Quarterly Review of Pediatrics*, VI (1951).

113. ———, and R. Rhines, *Spasticity, the Stretch Reflex and Extrapyramidal System* (Springfield: Charles C. Thomas, Publisher, 1947).

114. Marland, P. M., "A Plan of Therapy for Cerebral Palsy Based on Reflex Inhibition and Manual Facilitation of Speech," *Folia Phoniatrica*, VI (1954).

115. Mecham, M. J., M. J. Berko, and F. G. Berko, *Speech Therapy in Cerebral Palsy* (Springfield, Ill.: Charles C. Thomas, Publisher, 1960).

116. "Mother and Child: A Vast New Study," *The Johns Hopkins Magazine* (June 1959).

117. Miller, E., and G. B. Rosenfeld, "The Psychologic Evaluation of Children with Cerebral Palsy and Its Implications for Treatment," *Journal of Pediatrics*, XLI (1952).

118. Moorehouse, L. E., and J. M. Cooper, *Lifting and Carrying the C P in the Home* (New York: United Cerebral Palsy, n.d.).

119. Moyer, C., and A. J. Davis, eds., *Neurophysiology in the Treatment of Neuromuscular Function: Lectures by Margaret S. Rood* (Harrisburg: The Pennsylvania Society for Crippled Children and Adults, 1958). Mimeographed.

120. Myklebust, H. R., "Language Disorders in Children," in *Handbook of Speech Pathology*, ed. L. E. Travis (New York: Appleton-Century Crofts, Inc., 1957).

121. Mysak, E., "A Servo Model for Speech Therapy," *Journal of Speech and Hearing Disorders*, XXIV (1959).

122. ———, *Reflex Therapy in the Treatment of Cerebral Palsy* (New York: Bureau of Publications, Teachers College, Columbia University, 1963).

123. ———, "Significance of Neurophysiological Orientation to Cerebral Palsy Habilitation," *Journal of Speech and Hearing Disorders*, XXIV (1959).

124. ———, "Dysarthria and Oropharyngeal Reflexology: A Review," *Journal of Speech and Hearing Disorders*, XXVIII (1963).

125. *Nervous System*, Ciba Collection of Medical Illustrations (Summit, New Jersey: Ciba Pharmaceutical Products, Inc., 1953), I.

126. Osgood, C. E., *Contemporary Approaches to Cognition: a Behavioristic Analysis* (Cambridge: Harvard University Press, 1957).

127. Palmer, M., "Speech Disorders in Cerebral Palsy," *The Nervous Child*, VIII (1949).

128. ———, "Speech Therapy in Cerebral Palsy," *Journal of Pediatrics*, XL (1952).

129. ———, "Recent Advances in the Scientific Study of Language Disorders in Cerebral Palsy," *Cerebral Palsy Review*, XV (1954).

130. ———, "Studies in Clinical Techniques: Part III. Mandibular Facet Slip in Cerebral Palsy," *Journal of Speech and Hearing Disorders*, XIII (1948).

131. ———, "Laryngeal Blocks in Speech Disorders of Cerebral Palsy," *The Central States Speech Journal*, I (1949).

132. ———, "Studies in Clinical Techniques: Part II. Normalization of Chewing, Sucking and Swallowing Reflexes in Cerebral Palsy: A Home Program," *Journal of Speech Disorders*, XII (1947).

133. Patten, B. M., *Human Embryology*, 2nd ed. (New York, McGraw-Hill Book Company, 1953).

134. Penfield, W., *Speech and Brain Mechanisms* (Princeton, N. J.: Princeton University Press, 1959).

135. ———, and H. Japser, *Epilepsy and the Functional Anatomy of the Human Brain* (Boston: Little, Brown & Company, 1954).

136. ———, and T. Rasmussen, *The Cerebral Cortex of Man: A Clinical Study of Localization and Function* (New York: The Macmillan Company, 1950).

137. Perlstein, M. A., "Medical Aspects of Cerebral Palsy: Incidence, Etiology, Pathogenesis," *American Journal of Occupational Therapy*, IV (1950).

138. ———, "Infantile Cerebral Palsy, Classification and Clinical Correlations," *Journal of the American Medical Association*, CXLIX (1952).

139. ———, H. Barnett and J. Finder, *Therapeutic Equipment for Cerebral Palsied Children* (Chicago: The National Society for Crippled Children and Adults, 1953).

140. ———, E. L. Gibbs, and F. A. Gibbs, "The Electroencephalogram in Infantile Cerebral Palsy," *Proceedings of the Association for Research in Nervous and Mental Disease*, XXVI (1946).

141. Phelps, W. M., "Let's Define Cerebral Palsy," *Crippled Child*, XXVI (1948).

142. ———, "Bracing for Cerebral Palsy," *Crippled Child*, XX (1950).

143. ———, "Bracing in the Cerebral Palsies," in *Orthopedic Appliances Atlas* (Ann Arbor: J. W. Edwards, Inc., 1952), I.

144. ———, "The Treatment of the Cerebral Palsies, *Journal of Bone and Joint Surgery*, XXII (1940).

145. ———, "Factors Influencing the Treatment of Cerebral Palsy," *Physiotherapy Review*, XXI (1941).

146. Piaget, J., *The Origins of Intelligence in Children* (New York: International University Press, 1952).

147. Plotkin, W. H., "Situational Speech Therapy for Retarded Cerebral Palsied Children," *Journal of Speech and Hearing Disorders*, XXIV (1959).

148. Powdermaker, F., "Familial Congenital Spastic Diplegia," *American Journal of Diseases of Children*, XXXIX (1930).

149. *Realistic Educational Planning for Children with Cerebral Palsy* (New York: United Cerebral Palsy, 1951). A series of pamphlets covering pre-elementary through college level.

150. Robinault, I. P., "Perceptual Defects and Their Relationship to Therapy," *Cerebral Palsy Review*, XIX (1958).

151. Rood, M. S., "Neurophysiological Mechanisms Utilized in the Treatment of Neuromuscular Dysfunction," *American Journal of Occupational Therapy*, X (1956).

152. ———, "Neurophysiological Reactions as a Basis for Physical Therapy," *Physical Therapy Review*, XXXIV (1954).

153. Ruby, D. M., and W. D. Matheny, "Comments on Growth of Cerebral Palsied Children," *Journal of the American Dietetic Association*, XL (1962).

154. Rutherford, B. R., "Use of Negative Practice in Speech Therapy with

Children Handicapped by Cerebral Palsy, Athetoid Type," *Journal of Speech Disorders*, V (1940).

155. ———, *Give Them a Chance to Talk* (Minneapolis: Burgess Publishing Co., 1956).

156. ———, "Hearing Loss in Cerebral Palsied Children," *Journal of Speech Disorders*, X (1945).

157. Schacht, W. S., H. M. Wallace, M. Palmer, and B. Slater, "Ophthalmologic Findings in Children with Cerebral Palsy," *Pediatrics*, XIX (1957), Part I.

158. Schilder, P., *The Image and Appearance of the Human Body* (New York: International Universities Press, 1935).

159. Schlanger, B., "Environmental Influences on the Verbal Output of Mentally Retarded Children," *Journal of Speech and Hearing Disorders*, XIX (1954).

160. Schut, J. U., "Hereditary Ataxia. Clinical Study through Six Generations," *Archives of Neurology and Psychiatry*, LXIII (1950).

161. Semans, S., "Physical Therapy for Motor Disorders Resulting from Brain Damage," *Rehabilitation Literature*, XX (1959).

162. *Services for Children with Cerebral Palsy* (New York: American Public Health Association, 1955).

163. Shelton, R. L., "Therapeutic Exercise and Speech Pathology," *Asha*, V (1963).

164. Sherrington, C. S., *The Integrative Action of the Nervous System*, end ed. (New Haven: Yale University Press, 1947).

165. Shirley, M., *The First Two Years* (Minneapolis: University Minneasplis Press, 1933).

166. Shriner, M., *Foundations for Walking: A Practical Guide for Therapists, Teachers and Parents of Cerebral Palsied Children* (Chicago: The National Society for Crippled Children and Adults, 1951).

167. Snidecor, J. C., "The Speech Correctionist on the Cerebral Palsy Team," *Journal of Speech and Hearing Disorders*, XIII (1948).

168. Solomon, B., "Relation of Oral Sensation to Oral Motor Skills in Athetoids." Unpublished Doctoral Dissertation, The Pennsylvania State University, 1964.

169. Solomon, P. et. al., eds., *Sensory Deprivation* (Cambridge: Harvard University Press, 1961).

170. St. James, R., "Treatment of Cerebral Palsy," *Physical Therapy Review*, XXVIII (1948).

171. Stetson, R. H., *Motor Phonetics: A Study of Speech Movements in Action*, 2nd ed, (Amsterdam: North Holland Publishing Company, 1951).

172. Strauss, A. A., and N. C. Kephart, *Psycholopathology and Education of Brain Injured Children*, Progress in Theory and Clinic (New York: Grune & Stratton, Inc., 1955), II.

173. ———, and L. E. Lehtinen, *Psychopathology and Education of the Brain Injured Child* (New York: Grune & Stratton, Inc. 1951).

174. *Surveys of Cerebral Palsy* (New York: United Cerebral Palsy, 1955).

175. Swinyard, C. A., "Reflections about Reflex Therapy in Cerebral Palsy," *Physical Therapy Review*, XXXIX (1959).

176. Taylor, E. M., *Psychological Appraisal of Children with Cerebral Defects* (Cambridge, Harvard University Press, 1959).
177. Templin, M., *Certain Language Skills in Children* (Minneapolis: University of Minnesota Press, 1957).
178. *Thought in the Young Child: Report on a Conference on Intellective Development,* Monographs of the Society for Research in Child Development, XXVII, No. 2 (1962).
179. Tizard, J. P., R. S. Paine, and B. Crothers, "Disturbances of Sensation in Children with Hemiplegia," *Journal of the American Medical Association,* CLV (1954).
180. Van Riper, C., *Teaching Your Child to Talk* (New York: Harper & Row, Publishers, Inc., 1950).
181. ——, *Speech Correction: Principles and Methods,* 4th ed. (Englewood Cliffs, N. J.: Prentice-Hall, Inc., 1963).
182. von Bonin, G., *The Cerebral Cortex* (Springfield, Illinois: Charles C. Thomas, Publisher, 1960).
183. Wenger, M. A., F. N. Jones, and M. H. Jones, *Physiological Psychology* (New York: Holt, Rinehart & Winston, Inc., 1956).
184. Wepman, I. M., L. V. Jones, R. D. Bock, and D. V. Pelt, "Studies in Aphasia, Background and Theoretical Formulations," *Journal of Speech and Hearing Disorders,* XXV (1960).
185. West, R. E., ed., *Childhood Aphasia* (San Francisco: California Society for Crippled Children and Adults, 1962).
186. ——, M. Ansberry, and A. Carr, *The Rehabilitation of Speech,* 3rd ed. (New York, Harper & Row, Publishers, Inc., 1957).
187. Westlake, H., "Muscle Training for Cerebral Palsied Speech Cases," *Journal of Speech and Hearing Disorders,* XVI (1951).
188. ——, *A System for Developing Speech with Cerebral Palsied Children* (Chicago: The National Society for Crippled Children and Adults, 1951). Reprinted from the June, August, October, and December 1951 issues of *The Crippled Child.*
189. ——, and D. Rutherford, *Speech Therapy for the Cerebral Palsied* (Chicago: National Society for Crippled Children and Adults, 1961).
190. Wiedenbaker, R., M. Sandry, and G., Moed, "Sensory Discrimination of Children with Cerebral Palsy: Pressure-Pain Thresholds on the Foot," *Perceptual and Motor Skills,* XVII (1963).
191. Wood, Nancy E., *Language Disorders in Children* (Chicago: National Society for Crippled Children and Adults, 1959).
192. Wortis, H. Z., "Some Aspects of Parent-Child Relation in Cerebral Palsy," *Cerebral Palsy Review,* XV (1954).
193. Wright, B. A., *Physical Disability—A Psychological Approach* (New York: Harper & Row, Publishers, Inc., 1960).
194. Zubek, J. P., and L. Wilgosh, "Prolonged Immobilization of the Body: Changes in Performance and in the Electroencephalogram." *Science,* CXL (1963).
195. Zuk, G. H., "Perceptual Processes in Normal Development, Brain Injury and Mental Retardation," *American Journal of Mental Deficiency,* LXIII (1958).

index